Fundraising Skills for Health Care Executives

Joyce J. Fitzpatrick, PhD, RN, FAAN, is Elizabeth Brooks Ford Professor of Nursing at the Frances Payne Bolton School of Nursing, Case Western Reserve University (CWRU) where she was Dean of Nursing from 1982 through 1997. During her tenure as dean, the endowment of the school was increased from approximately $8.5 million to $50 million and the School obtained 10 endowed chairs for nursing. She provided the leadership for two capital campaigns for nursing; in the latter campaign the School of Nursing raised more than $26 million. Dr. Fitzpatrick is well known as an international scholar and leader in nursing.

Sandra S. Deller, BA, is Director of Major Gifts and Special Assistant to the Vice President for University Relations and Development, Case Western Reserve University. The University development team, of which she is a part, successfully raised $101.3M in total gifts and pledges in 1998–99. She has been a fundraising professional for 17 years. She led the CWRU School of Nursing development staff in two successful campaigns, first a campaign for critical care nursing in which $5.5M was raised, and a component of the University's $350M capital campaign in which the school of nursing raised over $26M. Ms. Deller is on the Board of the Greater Cleveland Chapter of the National Society of Fund Raising Executives.

Fundraising Skills for Health Care Executives

Joyce J. Fitzpatrick, PhD, RN, FAAN
Sandra S. Deller

 Springer Publishing Company

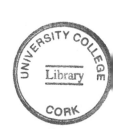

Springer Publishing Company, Inc.
536 Broadway
New York, NY 10012-3955

Acquisitions Editor: Sheri W. Sussman
Production Editor: Pamela Lankas
Cover design by Susan Hauley

00 01 02 03 04 / 5 4 3 2 1

Library of Congress Cataloging-in-Publication Data

Fundraising skills for health care executives / Joyce J. Fitzpatrick and Sandra S. Deller.
    p.   cm.
    Includes bibliographical references and index.
    ISBN 0-8261-1367-2
    1. Nursing schools—Endowments.   2. Medical education—Endowments.
3. Health facilities—Endowments.   4. Fund raising.   5. Fund raisers
(Persons).   I. Fitzpatrick, Joyce J., 1944–.   II. Deller, Sandra S.

RT73.F86 2000
362.1'068'1—dc21
                                                                00-058829

Printed in the United States of America

Contents

Contributors *vii*

Preface *ix*

1 Introduction 1
Joyce J. Fitzpatrick and Sandra S. Deller

2 History of Philanthropy 7
Joyce J. Fitzpatrick and Sandra S. Deller

3 Basic Principles of Development 11
Sandra S. Deller and Joyce J. Fitzpatrick

4 Types of Gifts, Ways of Giving, and Special
Fundraising Activities 24
Sandra S. Deller and Joyce J. Fitzpatrick

5 Reasons for Giving 38
Joyce J. Fitzpatrick and Sandra S. Deller

6 Individual Gifts 44
Joyce J. Fitzpatrick and Sandra S. Deller

7 Planned Giving 55
Duncan Hartley

8 Foundation and Corporate Development 76
Myrna J. Petersen

9 Volunteers and Committees for Fundraising 95
Joyce J. Fitzpatrick and Sandra S. Deller

10 Campaigns 103
Sandra S. Deller and Joyce J. Fitzpatrick

11 Stewardship and Recognition 113
Sandra S. Deller and Joyce J. Fitzpatrick

v

12   Case Studies   119
       Joyce J. Fitzpatrick and Sandra S. Deller

13   Staffing the Development Office and Other
       Organizational Issues   124
       Joyce J. Fitzpatrick and Sandra S. Deller

Appendices

A   Sample Gift Table   135

B   Resources and Bibliography for Fundraising   137

C   Endowed Chairs Articles   145

D   Fundraising Articles   157

E   Fundraising Reports from the Council for Aid to Education   167

Index   187

Contributors

Duncan Hartley
Assistant Vice President
University Relations and
    Development
and Head
Office of Gift Planning
Case Western Reserve University
Cleveland, OH

Myrna Petersen
Director Foundation and
    Corporate Relations
School of Nursing
University of Maryland
Baltimore, MD

Preface

Over the past 10 years we have received a number of requests from colleagues, primarily deans of schools of nursing, to provide consultation regarding fundraising. Although we consistently have communicated the fact that there is no magic, we also have shared the techniques and the processes that are embedded in successful efforts such as the one that we led at the Case Western Reserve University School of Nursing in the 1990s. There are many skills that can be taught, practiced, and implemented. Yet, fundraising remains at the core an interpersonal process.

Together we were able to capitalize on each other's strengths, and develop both the structures and processes to position the school of nursing as a positive force within the local, national, and global nursing community. The public relations aspect of our fundraising efforts was ever present, not only in the formal components of our work, but also in the informal communication and activities. Both our public relations and our fundraising endeavors were recognized. Through the campaign for the School of Nursing we successfully raised over $26 million, and positioned the School in the leadership role that it continues to enjoy in the nursing and health care environments.

We know that others laid the groundwork for the successes that we shared, including leaders within the university and school environment. And, as we have communicated in this book, we believe that everyone engaged in fundraising must assume a long-term perspective. Thus, we believe that we have planted the fundraising seeds for generations to come.

We present this book as a practical guide for the novice, as well as experienced deans and executives within health care institutions, and for the development officers within these organizations. We have described the strategies and activities that worked for us so that others can adapt them to their own challenges in fundraising. We encourage you to adapt them creatively, and to find the cadence in fundraising that works within your team and institution.

JOYCE J. FITZPATRICK
SANDRA S. DELLER

ix

1

Introduction

JOYCE J. FITZPATRICK AND SANDRA S. DELLER

Fundraising is rapidly becoming an expectation for executives in health science schools, particularly the largest and most prestigious schools. Deans of schools of nursing, medicine, and dentistry are expected to initiate and manage a wide range of development activities, often in concert with the universities and the health care institutions with which they have primary affiliations. Fundraising also is an expectation among key health care leaders in the service delivery arena. Many health care systems have extensive development departments and several fundraising staff members, just as the major private universities have large development departments.

No one prepares the new dean or health care executive for fundraising. Rather, it is one of the skills that is expected, but not explicitly taught. There is often an underlying belief that fundraising is something that anyone can do. At the same time that it is believed that there is nothing to learn about fundraising, the individual executive may have the attitude that "I could never ask anyone for money." Sometimes, deans or executives find themselves in the middle of a campaign before they realize that they need help. Consequently, there is great demand for consultants who might help with the fundraising process, for both new and experienced deans. Often, what the consultant communicates is very individual and informal. Based on our experience and successes in fundraising, we often have been asked to provide consultation to colleagues launching fundraising campaigns. Through this book, it is our goal to formalize and systematically communicate the key components of fundraising that we believe will lead to success. Much of the content included here is what we would share through the consultation process.

There are several myths and misperceptions about fundraising that we address in this book. The intent is to dispel the myths and to clarify the misperceptions. These common misunderstandings include:

1. There are no special skills that are required of the executive or any of the volunteers or staff involved in the fundraising.
2. The primary fundraising responsibility belongs to the development officer.
3. Fundraising will happen automatically if the academic and clinical programs are strong.
4. Fundraising is a special skill that is separate and apart from the mission of the organization.

Further, we build on basic principles of fundraising that have served us well in our collaborative development efforts. These include:

1. People give to people.
2. People give when there is vision; need alone is not sufficient.
3. People are more likely to give when asked.

We have tried to make explicit some of what we have learned during our collaborative fundraising experiences, and reassure the readers that there is no right way to go about raising money. There are, however, guidelines and principles that can be shared with others.

OUR FUNDRAISING EXPERIENCES

Together we have spent nearly 50 years of our combined professional careers in higher education. The majority of this time has been spent in private institutions in which there was a major emphasis on the fundraising responsibilities of deans, senior administrative officers and, of course, fundraising professionals (development officers). We first began our professional association as part of a team responsible for a capital campaign for one of the top schools of nursing in the nation. This multiyear professional relationship taught us much about the fundraising potential for schools of nursing, nursing organizations, other health science schools, and other health care institutions. A key component of our task was raising the visibility of nurses within the health care system and within the educational institutions. We learned that in the fundraising arena, as in many others, nurses are often not visible partners in the process of health care and education. We learned much about our own roles, and about the need to teach others like ourselves what executives in health care institutions often learn from "on the job" exposure to fundraising.

Most academic administrators are chosen for their scholarly contributions to the discipline and for their administrative skills. Only recently has there been attention to the need for academic administrators in nursing and health care to possess some fundraising skills in addition to their other skills. Yet, many of the same characteristics that make a good executive will make that executive a good fundraiser. Most critical among the qualities for the executive are the following: a commitment to the goals of the institution, good public speaking skills, i.e., the ability to translate the vision into a message for others, good interpersonal relationships and skills at interpersonal communication, a deep interest in other people, and a willingness to help and to lead. Many of these same skills are necessary for the fundraising professional, the development officer who will participate with the executive to achieve the fundraising goals. Yet, these skills must be complementary; one professional must enhance the functioning of the other.

As we were most successful with our capital campaign, raising over $26 million for the school of nursing in approximately 5 years, we began receiving many requests from leaders within other institutions, particularly schools of nursing, to consult with them. What we discovered in our discussions with others is that many of our colleagues were eager to learn about fundraising, but needed some basic information in order to proceed. Also, there were some consistent misperceptions that we thought were important to clarify. For example, many deans were unclear about the central role that they had to play in the fundraising activity, preferring to hire professional fundraisers to complete the task. Also, there continues to be a great deal of misperception about the ease with which one can raise endowment funds. Most deans did not understand the development process as a long-term investment. Yet it is clear to us that many of the benefits of our efforts in the capital campaign that we concluded in the mid-1990s will be reaped by our successors. For development is literally a process of "planting the seeds," nurturing the relationships, and growing the results.

We believe that our development efforts were successful largely because of our team effort, our willingness to learn from each other, to take risks together, and to build on our basic skills of comfort in interpersonal interactions, our flexibility, and our ability to "think on our feet." But, there is no question; if we were to identify the one most critical factor in our success, it would be our sincere interest in other people. We were successful in raising money because we developed strong interpersonal relationships with the potential donors. We cared about each of them, and worked very diligently to determine ways in which we could help them achieve their goals while making a financial contribution to the School of Nursing.

Through our collaborative fundraising efforts, all of our skills were challenged. It was an intensive time when we needed to be consciously and constantly "on call" for the next opportunity and fundraising adventure. We worked together to achieve the defined goals for our campaign, and grew to understand each other's strengths and competencies in the development process. We became known for our collective spirit in the institution where we worked, and the community where we worked and lived. There was never any doubt in the potential prospects' minds, at least as far as we were aware, of the total commitment that we had to the institution and to the goals of the School of Nursing. We believed totally in our product, and thus, were able to sell it to others.

Through sharing our "lessons learned" we hope to set the stage for more extensive discussion of fundraising for nursing and health care, particularly among the executives and the fundraising staff within schools of nursing, other health science schools, and other health care organizations. In this brief text, we have included the majority of key topics in the development literature. The text is meant as an introduction to the process of fundraising, one that will serve as an orientation for new deans or health care executives, or deans or executives who are new to the fundraising process.

We have included the basics of fundraising among individuals and foundations and corporations. Also, we have attended to the specifics of fundraising during campaigns and the special components of fundraising for planned gifts. Most of all we have shared with the readers our strategies for success, whether in the design and implementation of structures for supporting the development activities in the school of nursing or health care institution, or through our discussion of the case studies that we have selected to profile in chapter 12.

Throughout the book we try to clarify several misperceptions about fundraising. We also try to make the fundraising process simplistic and understandable so that it can be implemented without much difficulty.

Because we have worked closely together as a team, and because that work was very successful, we have included the ideas of both the development officer and the dean or executive throughout the book. Each chapter includes the special perspective of the development officer and the dean or executive. We think that this relationship should be complementary in all activities having to do with fundraising.

DEVELOPMENT OFFICER'S PERSPECTIVE

It is not only important, but also critical, that the development officer and dean have good chemistry. The perception of them as a team helps to build fundraising confidence. We were fortunate to work well together and blend styles so flawlessly that on solicitation calls a cue could be picked up and a conversation steered to another priority that was closer to the prospect's interests.

Other important ingredients of this fundraising collaboration are trust and tenaciousness. The dean has to delegate appropriate authority to his/her development officer. On certain occasions and with certain activities, the development officer needs to have the authority to speak for the dean and to interpret the dean's vision for the organization. A component of that trust is some control over the dean's calendar and time. It is a given that a certain percentage of the dean's time to visit or call major prospects needs to be allocated for fundraising. In a campaign, this time can be substantial.

The dean can set the expectation with the potential donor that the development officer will follow up the request and address questions. This validates the development officer's follow-up and frees the dean for other responsibilities. If the solicitation becomes stalled or if major policy issues arise, the dean needs to be apprised of these obstacles so appropriate action can be taken and the objective achieved.

Talking to other deans, we found that one of the fundraising stumbling blocks was raising sights for "asks." Some seemed timid about asking for too much. As we will discuss, there are more stories of money "left on the table" by too conservative a request. Prospects are not alienated by too large an "ask."

A few deans are simply not comfortable with making "the ask." The development officer can assume that role. To make the request effective, usually the dean describes the vision and needs of the organization; after this description, the development officer makes the request, naming the amount to realize the dean's objectives.

In this book, we hope to demonstrate that this collaboration for fundraising can be exhilarating. The rewards are many for the institution and for the individuals involved in meeting outstanding individuals. The pace and pressure, too, can be exciting. Remember to enjoy it. Fundraising can be fun. Making it a positive experience attracts others who want to join a winning team.

DEAN OR EXECUTIVE'S PERSPECTIVE

Our positive experiences with fundraising were no doubt due to the camaraderie that we shared, and also to the value that we placed on fundraising in relation to the strategic plan for the institution. And many donors told us that the enthusiasm that our team communicated was an important factor in their decision to give. Yet, it is important not to confuse the messenger with the message. Our message about the school was always clear and targeted toward important educational goals. There was never any ambiguity in the message, and there was never a sense that we were only fundraising for the sake of generating funds or accumulating funds. This is important to note, as many donors expect integrity in the development process, and become angry and disappointed when they feel used. It is never acceptable to be "less than truthful" in fundraising. All individuals expect more from the leadership of health care institutions.

Another characteristic of our collaborative success was the drive and determination that we had to "tell our story." Often, we would find that major prospects knew little about the School of Nursing or the contributions of nurse leaders, particularly compared to medical education and contributions. Enhancing the visibility of the School and "friend-raising" among new constituents became extremely important in our long-range planning.

SUMMARY

We hope that we have communicated to the reader the fact that there is no right or wrong way to fundraise. Key ingredients for success for development officers and health care executives include the link to the strategic plan, the consistency between the vision and the plan, and the honesty and integrity of the process.

2

History of Philanthropy

Joyce J. Fitzpatrick and Sandra S. Deller

GENERAL HISTORY OF PHILANTHROPY
IN THE UNITED STATES

American philanthropy can trace its beginnings to 1630, when John Winthrop preached "A Model of Christian Charity" to Puritans bound for territory that would eventually become New England. In 1638, John Harvard bequeathed his library and half of his estate to a newly founded school in Cambridge, Massachusetts, which now bears his name. Scientist, printer, and statesman, Benjamin Franklin, was one of the most successful fundraisers of the late 18th and early 19th centuries. He used special prospect lists and personal calls to found a hospital, a university, America's first free library, a church, and a volunteer fire department.

In fact, two of the world's noblest institutions, the hospital and the university, evolved through private funding. Universities and health care institutions have long been favorites among donors wishing to endow institutions and to invest in either good works, through the health care institutions, or in the generations of the future, through the universities. And, of course, churches have consistently relied on donors for their revenues.

Many famous philanthropists are well known in American history, as much for their philanthropic endeavors as for their business acumen. These include John D. Rockefeller, who gave $600,000 in 1889 to found the University of Chicago; his son, John D. Rockefeller, Jr. who financed the restoration of Williamsburg, Virginia in 1927 and donated 17 acres of land in Manhattan for the United Nations Headquarters in 1946; and Andrew Carnegie, whose will commitment in 1919 totaled $350 million in contributions. Contemporary philanthropists of the same level would include Bill Gates and Ted Turner, both of whom have made substantial gifts in the past 5 years.

The profession of fundraising in the United States began in the last decade of the 19th century with the efforts of Lyman Pierce and Charles Ward. Pierce was financial membership secretary of the YMCA in Omaha, and Ward was undersecretary of the YMCA in Grand Rapids. Pierce invented the concept of the campaign; he enlisted volunteers in his efforts, divided them into teams, prepared and printed materials and held regular meetings with the volunteers.

RECENT STATISTICS RELATED TO EDUCATION

During 1998, private contributions to America's colleges and universities increased significantly. According to the Council for Aid to Education's (CAE) May 1999 report, total contributions rose 15% over the 1997 level of $16 billion. Total gift income during the 1997 academic year (July 1996 through June 1997) was estimated at $16 billion, a $1.75 billion increase over the 1996 academic year figures. Private support to higher education has risen steadily in the 1990s; in 1998 contributions were 64% greater than in 1993. (Copies of significant CAE charts are included in Appendix A.)

Two major factors were cited by CAE as contributing to the increases for 1997 and 1998. These included the increase in gifts for capital purposes and the overall healthy state of the economy as measured by the Gross Domestic Product (GDP), which historically has shown a close correlation to gifts for current operations of academic institutions.

During 1998, all sources increased their giving, including alumni, nonalumni contributors, corporations, foundations, and religious and other organizations. Contributions from alumni accounted for 30% of the gifts; nonalumni individual gifts (including those of parents) accounted for 24%; corporations 18%; foundations 21%; and religious and other organizations contributed 8% of the total. Over the past 20 years the most significant increases in giving have been from alumni. Their giving has increased by 157% in the 20-year period (CAE Press Release, 1999).

A recent report of the American Association of Fund Raising Counsel (AAFRC) Trust for Philanthropy indicated that charitable giving reached a record-breaking $175 billion in 1998, up 10% from 1997 (AAFRC, 1999). Giving in all four categories studied, including individuals, bequests, foundations, and corporations, all showed healthy increases. As has been the case for years, individuals (and their bequests) yield the largest amount in gifts. In 1998, individuals and their bequests accounted for approximately 85% of the gifts.

Of particular interest to Schools of Nursing, but relevant to all fundraising efforts, are the current statistics regarding women and wealth. Currently, women own about 75% of America's stocks and bonds and 65% of the savings accounts, and own or control 70% of the country's capital. In addition to all of this, women control more than 85% of consumer buying power. Thus, it is important not to underestimate the power of women in fundraising. As women live approximately 8 years longer than men, and have fought recently to gain financial power, they have changed the landscape of fundraising activities. In particular, estate planning for women has received much emphasis, and should be highlighted in any campaign.

SCHOOLS OF NURSING AS AN EXAMPLE OF THE CHANGE IN HIGHER EDUCATION

In 1923, as a result of significant philanthropic gifts, schools of nursing were begun in three private universities. These were Vanderbilt University, Western Reserve University (now Case Western Reserve University), and Yale University. In these private schools of nursing, as well as in many others, fundraising is an important component of the dean's role. These three schools of nursing continue to be among the most heavily endowed among all schools of nursing. Although there has not been an effort to determine overall endowment or fundraising statistics among schools of nursing, the information obtained since 1984 regarding endowed chairs in schools of nursing gives a glimpse into the levels of endowments for chairs and professorships. When the first survey was completed in 1984, only 20 chairs were identified in schools of nursing (Fitzpatrick, 1985). In the update of the endowed chairs article, published in January 2000, 167 endowed chairs and professorships were identified (Fitzpatrick, 2000). This phenomenal growth in endowed chairs is a result of several factors, including the enhanced visibility of schools of nursing within universities, the increase in fundraising skills among nursing school deans, and, more recently, the robust economy.

Capital campaigns also are now more common in schools of nursing, often with overall goals at the level of $15 million to $25 million. Full time development staff within schools of nursing are now more commonplace, particularly at the private schools of nursing, but also among the public institutions with major development programs. In our successful campaign at the Case Western Reserve University School of Nursing, the goal was $15 million. We exceeded the goal and raised $26 million over a 5-year period.

REFERENCES

AAFRC Press Release. (1999, May 25). *Total giving increased 10.7% in 1998*. http://www.aafrc.org

CAE Press Release. (1999, May 28). *Private contributions to higher education soar to record breaking levels*. http://www.cae.org

Fitzpatrick, J. J. (1985). Endowed chairs in nursing: State of the art. *Journal of Professional Nursing, 1*, 145–147.

Fitzpatrick, J. J. (2000). A 1999 update on endowed chairs and professorships in schools of nursing. *Journal of Professional Nursing, 16*, 57–62.

3

Basic Principles of Development

SANDRA S. DELLER AND JOYCE J. FITZPATRICK

Three aspects of the basic development process are discussed in this chapter: research in identifying and rating prospects, cultivation of prospects, and solicitation of potential donors. All three components are equally important in a successful fundraising effort.

RESEARCH

Research is the foundation of a successful development campaign. By identifying potential donors or prospects through research, an institution ensures that its development resources will be focused on individuals of influence and affluence. While larger institutions often maintain a research staff or department to track prospects, an organization of a smaller size can use basic indicators such as relationship to the institution, financial status, age, marital status, education, and business information to determine giving potential.

Research should begin with the individuals who are closest to the institution. Board members, committee members, and interested community leaders are key prospects for most institutions. Colleges and universities count faculty, alumni, and their families as primary prospects. Additionally, grateful patients should be considered. In any development campaign, the individuals most likely to participate and ultimately become supporters will be those with a past or current association with the institution.

Past contributions and current associations are significant criteria for gauging a prospect's potential for supporting the development initiative.

11

Institutions that conduct an annual fund drive should study past campaigns over a period of years, if possible, and document both donors who made significant contributions and repeat donors. To determine potential based on association, the institution should consider the length and strength of the relationship by investigating the origin and nature of the association and any history of family involvement. Familiar board members, staff, and faculty may provide insight into the current or future contribution potential of past donors and individuals associated with the institution.

Other critical indicators of giving potential include salary, net worth, family background, individually or family owned businesses, club memberships, real estate holdings, hobbies, and collections. In selecting prospects for development, the institution should weigh these criteria against financial obligations. Children, grandchildren, and older parents who require support for their living expenses or health care affect the resources available for philanthropy.

The prospect's age and marital status are also important considerations. There may not be sufficient time to cultivate successful relationships with elderly prospects. Some elderly individuals are very reluctant to make changes to their estate plans once they feel their affairs are in order. Some younger prospects who are still accumulating wealth may require years to reach the stage where philanthropic contributions become a viable consideration. Conversely, individuals who are no longer in the acquisitive mode and have never married, or are widowed, often wish to leave some legacy and are, therefore, excellent long or short-term prospects. There are always exceptions: each prospect should be carefully evaluated.

From the individuals who are likely to support a development campaign, the institution should select a manageable number of prospects for solicitation. Depending on the institutional requirements and size of the development staff, this can vary from 100 to 150 prospects per development professional.

THE DEVELOPMENT OFFICER'S PERSPECTIVE

As a development professional for a university, I look first and foremost to relationships when considering new prospects: how long, and how strong. Because the primary prospects are most often alumni, I look for "selling points"; for example the anniversary of graduation is often a time of nostalgia. Campaigns provide a motivation, and the time line is a convenient impetus to close a gift. Relevance of career or hobbies to educational initiatives provides information along with indicators of wealth and propensity to give. In planning the approach, I consider the individual's age as well as the existence of dependents or obligations that impact the ability to give. Opportunities to honor a loved one can be a powerful incentive.

THE DEAN'S PERSPECTIVE

The dean and faculty represent a key link for potential donors. The key academic leaders can help to identify donors whose interests mesh with the current programs and activities, as well as new aspects of programmatic initiatives built into the strategic plan.

Every opportunity should be used in gathering information about the interests of alumni and potential donors, and good records should be kept. The research database is crucial to all fundraising efforts.

INFORMATION RESOURCES

In order to select the most promising prospects, the institution should compile individual profiles that estimate potential for giving. These profiles should describe the source of wealth along with all known financial resources and holdings. Publications such as *Who's Who, Standard and Poor's,* and *Who's Wealthy in America* and World Wide Web sites for the *Wall Street Journal, Fortune,* and *Forbes* are valuable resources for financial information. (For more information, see Internet resources in Appendix B.)

When compiling a profile on individuals whose wealth is associated with corporations, the institution should research the corporation where the prospect works or has ownership. Other corporate trustee appointments, such as board memberships, provide a source of income or stock, as well as a potential eligibility for matching gifts as trustee. Individuals whose wealth is associated with a public company can be profiled using annual reports, stock prices, and analytical forecasts, since these are required to be released to the public. One World Wide Web resource is http://www.edgar-online.com, which is an easily searchable site that provides free corporate proxies and other government filings.

For prospects associated with private companies, gift potential is more difficult to ascertain, as the company is not required to disclose financial data. The individuals themselves, or their business associates, are often the best resources for information in compiling financial profiles. In addition, many companies, both public and private, maintain web pages, which can be accessed by using a search engine. Though the information contained on these sites is self-reported and usually focused toward marketing, corporate web pages often include financial statements and descriptions of key executives and company products that are a valuable resource in compiling a prospect's profile.

Individuals whose source of wealth is through family are often associated with philanthropic foundations. Family foundations must file a tax return (990) annually with the Internal Revenue Service. These individuals can be profiled using tax returns and information available through the Foundation Center, a significant development resource. (Additional information on the Foundation Center can be found in Appendix B. There are five field offices for the Center, including major sites in New York City, Washington, DC, Atlanta, San Francisco, and Cleveland. Their web site is http://www.Fdncenter.com.)

Information on individual property holdings is available through the County Assessor's Office. Though this data is sometimes only available by written or personal request, a telephone call can usually verify whether the prospect owns the property. Real estate offices can also provide information concerning the approximate property value of a prospect's residence by indicating a high and low for home sales in a specific neighborhood.

Outside development consultants also can be used to screen data for prospects based on criteria such as residency in upscale neighborhoods, business titles, board memberships, possessions such as luxury cars or boats, and even magazine subscriptions. Consultants will analyze data to project a prospect's resources and propensity to give. The institution should review any data provided by outside consultants and prioritize prospects according to institutional requirements.

Surveys, focus groups, or screening groups provide additional resources for profiling prospects. Screening groups comprised of affluent individuals who are close to the institution are most often used prior to the commencement of a campaign. Group members review a list of prospects and rate them according to motivations for giving, such as familiarity with the institution, and maximum propensity for giving, providing a gauge for "ask" amounts and information on potential campaign volunteers. An added benefit is the increased awareness of the participants of their own financial commitment.

CULTIVATION

Cultivation is an integral aspect in establishing a foundation for the solicitation or "ask." Cultivation activities increase awareness and interest and, if executed properly, can enhance the prospect's appreciation of the institution, sparking a commitment to contribution.

Activities that constitute cultivation are sometimes categorized as direct or indirect moves. Direct moves include phone calls and personal visits, including breakfast, lunch, or dinner meetings. Securing an appointment to execute a direct or foreground move should not be difficult for prospects closely associated with the institution. It is, however, a crucial step when reaching out to lesser known prospects.

A peer or friend of the prospect who is available and willing to participate can be a catalyst to open the lines of communication. The development professional, however, should not wait for the perfect peer to volunteer before making contact. Development staff should request appointments with a level of confidence that suggests that the appointment is secure and that the call is merely a confirmation of a convenient meeting time and place; new development staff might take some cues from telemarketers, who are trained to communicate and draw contacts into conversation, to hone their approach. The prospect's assistant will most likely be the first point of contact, and, as the prospect's appointment gatekeeper, should always be treated with respect. If engaged on a personal level, the assistant may be able to suggest the best times for reaching the prospect and perhaps even serve as an advocate to encourage a meeting. Some techniques are covered in the article in Appendix D: *Primer for Philanthropy: The ABC's of Fundraising*.

Research should provide an overview of the prospect that will be useful in securing an appointment. If research fails to supply useful information for demonstrating a knowledge of the prospect, the development professional may suggest familiarity with the prospect by using the individual's first name with the assistant; stockbrokers often circumvent the assistant or gatekeeper by using this technique. Referencing peers or friends of the prospect who have given permission to use their names for the contact is preferable.

In the case of individuals who are community leaders or top executives without an established relationship to the institution, it may be necessary for the institution's key executive personally to call to arrange the appointment. If the individual is a referral from a volunteer, reference this first. Sometimes volunteers may place the call. Unless you are certain the contact is going to occur with a sense of urgency, it is advisable to maintain control and initiate the contact from the institution's representative. Keep in mind that priorities and timelines often differ; also, some individuals overstate the nature of their relationships with important individuals.

In securing an appointment, the development professional should consider an appropriate meeting place. This will be dictated by the institution's resources and the prospect's preferences. If travel is feasible, the development professional should offer to visit the prospect. The alternative is an invitation for the prospect to visit the institution. Where appropriate, the development professional should allow the prospect to choose whether the meeting will incorporate a meal, or take place at the prospect's home or office. Personal visits can include peer volunteers and key representatives such as deans, directors of the institution, or favorite faculty or staff members, and incorporate a briefing on a topic of interest to the prospect. Initial meetings are first and foremost "discovery missions" in which listening is more important than talking. An experienced development officer should be present at these meetings to facilitate a comfortable relationship with the prospect and gather information for planning and initiating the solicitation.

Indirect moves include invitations to attend special group lectures or events. A prospect visiting the campus for such an engagement may be open to participating in a more intimate meeting organized to further cultivation.

In our experience we were successful in using several indirect techniques. The school enlisted the assistance of prospects for recruiting and marketing efforts and invited senior alumni prospects to share their educational and career experience at a forum including students and faculty. Some students also interviewed older alumni for an oral history project. To cultivate relationships with leaders in the field of nursing, the school invited prospects to speak as guest lecturers at classes and mentor students. The school complemented its indirect approach by developing an insider's newsletter to profile key prospects, donors, and innovative initiatives.

Whether cultivation activities are executed through direct or indirect moves, they should be designed to enhance the prospect's identity with and excitement regarding the institution and promote anticipation for future contacts.

THE DEVELOPMENT OFFICER'S PERSPECTIVE

The Development Officer should manage the process, plan the moves, and decide who should be involved and what activity is most effective in moving the prospect toward a solicitation. Research results, and any extraneous information gleaned from faculty or staff familiar with the prospect, will help to enhance the prospect's profile as preparation for a meeting or solicitation.

A personal visit is the preferred contact. Even if a personal visit requires travel, it is often the key to a successful solicitation. If time or budget constraints prohibit a personal visit, telephone calls are the next best approach to establishing and maintaining a relationship. The development officer or a key contact should place the calls at regular intervals. The conversation need not be lengthy; a call to touch base should be enough to keep the prospect's interest alive. Topics of conversation can include items discussed in the last call, including forthcoming vacations, anniversaries, or weddings or graduations in the prospect's family.

The conversation can then segue into a discussion concerning activities at the institution that might be of interest to the prospect, including major conferences, colloquiums involving faculty, or awards. College or university development staff might also provide updates on enrollment or recruitment statistics.

Between telephone calls, development staff should continue cultivation by sending the prospect news stories or clippings concerning the institution or subjects in which the prospect has expressed an interest. In addition, and where appropriate, development staff could send a feature story on the prospect to the institution's publication or invite the prospect to host a special event or activity. The time between personal contacts can be bridged with a myriad of cultivation activities; development personnel should always be alert to activities that strengthen the prospect's relationship with the institution.

THE DEAN'S PERSPECTIVE

It is extremely important for the dean to be available to the development staff at all times. In particular, the individual who has primary responsibility for managing fundraising should be the closest person to the dean, in relation to scheduling of important telephone calls and appointments. The dean must have a development officer who can help manage time, energy, resources, and activities around fundraising. Much of the success of fundraising, as with many other activities, is timing. Often, the request to a donor must be time-sensitive. Delaying fundraising activities in favor of academic projects is easy, especially when you are just learning the development business. If you do not have experience with fundraising, I would strongly recommend that you select an experienced fundraiser for the key development position.

SOLICITATION

As with sales, 80% of the money generated by development comes from 20% of the prospects solicited; people give to people. In the for-profit sector, several dealers sell the same makes and models of products, especially automobiles, for essentially the same price. A consumer's decision to buy at a particular dealership is based not on the dealer's product, but on the individual salesperson. So too in development; personnel and personal relationships are often the deciding factor in a prospect's decision to contribute to a particular institution. If the relationship is well developed, the prospect will want to find an excuse to give.

If cultivation activities are executed successfully, the prospect will feel an attachment to the institution. This relationship, however, does not automatically result in a donation. A successful solicitation requires an appeal not only to the prospect's relationship to the institution, but to the prospect as an individual.

Before the solicitation, development staff should review all research on the prospect, including contact reports and any history of donations. The next step is to select participants for the solicitation team. The individual who most frequently contacted the prospect should be present, if this is not the development officer. The development officer should be included to facilitate follow-up with the potential donor. Other participants might include key administrators, favorite faculty, trustees, or peer volunteers; the size of the "ask" and importance of the prospect dictates the appropriate number of participants involved in the solicitation.

The solicitation strategy should provide the most compelling case for supporting an identified institutional need that fits the prospect's interest and priorities. This approach is sometimes classified as the "marketing equation" or "exchange." Such a strategy requires the solicitors to place themselves in the role of the prospect. The solicitation should concentrate on those aspects of the project that are most important to the prospect's value set and the benefits or features that are most likely to inspire a contribution.

To help in developing the selection strategy, development staff and solicitor participants should recall past occasions of contact, focusing on the prospect's nonverbal communications as well as conversations for clues to prospect affinity. Body language such as a head nod indicates that the prospect is interested or excited about a subject. If seated, a movement forward indicates the solicitation has touched a nerve. Such "buying signals" reflected in nonverbal communication are sometimes more reliable than verbal communication in gauging the prospect's level of commitment.

Briefing sessions that bring contacts and peers together to discuss proposed strategies are advisable prior to major gift solicitations. This allows the development officer to take the lead in planning, organizing, and assisting in executing the solicitation while remaining open to other perspectives and ideas.

Participant briefing sessions should discuss who will make the solicitation and how to build toward it. A role-playing exercise is often helpful in these meetings to rehearse approaches to phrasing the request and potential outcomes. An optional strategy or fallback plan should also be developed during these sessions for initial requests that are not met with resounding enthusiasm. If a prospect responds that a gift at the level requested is not feasible, the solicitor should be prepared to request a leadership gift to the annual fund or a percentage increase on previous gifts.

In solicitation, flexibility is imperative. The solicitation team should prepare for the unexpected, assess the prospect's reactions, and be ready to readjust to address the prospect's interests and ensure the best opportunity for contribution.

The site selected for the solicitation can influence the outcome. Prospects often prefer to meet at locations that are comfortable for them, such as their home, office, social club, or favorite restaurant. The location selected should be conducive to conversation; noise levels are a factor when meeting in a public place, especially if the prospect is older. If the prospect agrees to meet at the institution, development staff should arrange for a comfortable room or office and convenient parking to ensure that the solicitation begins on a pleasant note. If you want the older prospect to review a proposal, be certain it is in larger print with sufficient white space.

Development staff should determine whether the prospect has any time constraints when scheduling the solicitation. Solicitors should remain conscious of this schedule, keeping the meeting as brief as possible, even if the prospect is retired or did not express any scheduling constraints. Prompt attendance by all solicitation participants is also important; the solicitors should always attempt to arrive at the site before the prospect. If the meeting includes dining, a comfortable seating arrangement is essential. The key solicitor should sit next to a prospect with a hearing disability or, otherwise, across from the prospect to promote eye contact. Before the meal, a solicitor may ask the waitstaff to delay taking the order so that the discussion and solicitation can progress. Likewise, if the meeting place is not at a private club, a solicitor may present a credit card to the restaurant in private before the meal to avoid any awkwardness at the meeting's conclusion. When ordering, solicitors should avoid foods that could present an embarrassment; lettuce tends to stick in the teeth, and foods that are difficult to manipulate, such as shellfish, could inadvertently jump to the prospect's plate or lap.

Since the decision to "buy" is usually made within the first 10 minutes of a solicitation, solicitors should begin the meeting by expressing the institution's appreciation for the prospect's counsel, involvement on committees, or past support, and by thanking the prospect for the opportunity to present a proposal. After reaffirming the prospect's interest in the future well-being of the institution, the solicitor can present the case for contribution. The solicitation should be a clear request for a gift of a specific amount and should explain how the gift will benefit the prospect or match the prospect's needs. Solicitors should balance the needs of the prospect with those of the institution, favoring proposals that are closest to the prospect's heart while avoiding proposals or gifts that do not advance the institution.

The type of gift will dictate the delivery of the solicitation. A solicitation for a scholarship might emphasize that the prospect relied on similar support to reach his or her current position. Memorial gifts, gifts that recognize a family member, or endowments should be described as a living legacy, while capital gifts can be recognized with a plaque or special signage.

The solicitor should emphasize the gift's impact on the institution, rather than its size, but should not be intimidated to request a significant sum or stretch gifts. Most prospects are flattered by such a solicitation, and, if asked for a smaller amount, might conclude that the solicitor did not adequately assess their resources. After making the request, the solicitor should remain silent until the prospect responds, taking careful note of the prospect's verbal and nonverbal cues and making certain to understand any objections and conditions for a future gift. If the gift is smaller than anticipated, the solicitor might offer options for paying over a period of years, ask if the gift could be considered as an initial payment, or suggest a planned gift. These requests should be made with sensitivity to avoid an impression that the gift's value is determined by its size. Before adjourning, the solicitor should summarize the meeting and discuss next steps.

ANSWERING OBJECTIONS

The solicitor often reacts to an objection with a racing pulse and sweaty palms, assessing the need to answer and overcome the objection as an obstacle to institutional objectives. An objection, however, can provide an opportunity to maximize potential results. In sales, this principle is described by the expression: "The sale begins with the first refusal." So too in development: An objection that is explored properly can provide the clues to a successful solicitation. When met with an objection, therefore, solicitors should remain calm, giving no indication of disappointment or irritation, and approaching it instead as an opener to the gift.

Objections sometimes arise due to incorrect assumptions and misidentification of the prospect's objectives. Preparation, therefore, is integral to answering and overcoming objections. The cultivation process should reveal areas of concern that need to be addressed before the prospect feels comfortable enough to commit resources. In addition, solicitors should explore potential objections and answers prior to the solicitation. Cash flow issues can be addressed by offering options for giving over a period of years. Likewise, a planned gift can serve the institution while providing income to the prospect's family, where objections are based on conflicting financial commitments to the prospect's parents or children. By identifying alternatives to giving that are tailored to the prospect's circumstances and estate-planning objectives, the solicitors may open the door to a larger gift than anticipated. Additionally, it signals a genuine interest in the prospect's needs.

Reviewing objections and preparing appropriate responses reduces the chance for surprise during the solicitation. Armed with proper preparation, the solicitor who listens and understands the prospect can begin the process of overcoming objections and pave the way to a successful solicitation.

DETERMINING THE REAL OBJECTION

To overcome objections, the solicitor must create an environment of trust in which the prospect feels comfortable to freely discuss his or her financial situation, philanthropic objectives, and resources. Open-ended questions promote more communication than questions that can be answered with a "yes" or "no." The solicitor can present an open-ended question by restating the prospect's objection with a statement such as "You seem concerned about preserving your estate for your family," or asking an indirect question to help clarify the objection.

Rephrasing techniques demonstrate the solicitor's recognition of the prospect's concerns. Through reiteration, the solicitor can also confirm his or her understanding of the prospect's objections. The process of restating and confirming the objection allows the prospect to further explain and clarify the objection and promotes a climate that is conductive to a collaborative solution. A solicitor speaking to a physician who is selling his or her practice might say, "We understand that you are selling your practice, that your cash flow is limited until that occurs, and that you are, therefore, uncomfortable committing to a contribution for this fiscal year." This sets the stage for a discussion of alternatives or appropriate dates to meet again and revisit the proposal. Alternatives may bring new objections, and the process should continue until both the prospect and solicitor agree upon the future direction of the relationship.

DEVELOPMENT OFFICER'S PERSPECTIVE

The development officer should view the process of overcoming objections as a challenge and an opportunity to close the gift. It provides the context for the next step and should help to define the most appropriate method and timetable for follow-up. If the team of solicitors has addressed all objections and done their best to provide creative alternatives and solutions, the prospect will usually be more willing to contribute. For example, prospects who are averse to relinquishing control of their money, such as entrepreneurs and family business owners, may be more willing to contribute to an interim proposal such as an annual fund or a gift distributed over a period of years. If the prospect still expresses reluctance, the development officer should ask what it would take to make the prospect comfortable enough to make the contribution.

THE DEAN OR EXECUTIVE'S PERSPECTIVE

As with other activities, fundraising requires being prepared. The more information and knowledge that you have about the prospect, including his or her interests and background, the more successful you will be in the fundraising.

Fundraising is built on knowledge: The knowledge that you can gain about the prospect through research and a series of interactions with the individual, knowledge of the institution and the match between institutional goals and donor desires, and knowledge of the various opportunities and types of fundraising, all matched to the donor's background and resources.

4

Types of Gifts, Ways of Giving, and Special Fundraising Activities

SANDRA S. DELLER AND JOYCE J. FITZPATRICK

This chapter is focused on the structures of gift giving that typically are used by institutions engaged in fundraising. Descriptions of the annual fund, challenge gifts, unrestricted and restricted funds, outright gifts, and bequests are included. Fundraising through direct-mail campaigns and special events also are addressed. Gift giving through campaigns is treated as a special category and described in chapter 10. Also, an entire chapter, chapter 7, is devoted to types of planned gifts.

ANNUAL FUND

Annual Fund gifts are the foundation of a giving pyramid. An Annual Fund is a yearly drive to solicit unrestricted funds that the institution can use for operations or for a particular need. Often the solicitation occurs around the close of the fiscal year or runs for one calendar year, then the process begins again.

The prospect base should consist of all existing donors, friends, and trustees. Additional prospects should be added through conversations with some of the key members of the existing annual donor group. Consider adding the names of any attendees of events. To be more effective in the appeal a chair or chairs of the Annual Fund Campaign should be recruited. If it is a school, members of all classes should be solicited preferably by a prominent classmate.

The key to Annual Fund success is to segment donors and develop gift clubs or gift levels. There is usually a perk or membership benefit for each level of gifting. This provides a rationale for asking individuals to consider joining or moving up to the next level, for example, the President's Society or the Founder's Society. Consider using a name of some distinguished leader or donor who was integral to your institution's success.

After analyzing the level of gifts received in past appeals, create the Gift Clubs to provide some incentive to increase giving. For example, if the largest gift secured has been at the $1000 level, you might want to add a $5000 club to give your $1000 donors an opportunity to expand their philanthropy. Gift clubs' benefits are modest at the lower end; at the lower end, it might just be a listing in a newsletter. The next gift level should be given a more prominent entry and an invitation to a special conference or activity. These donors could be sent special bulletins from the institution or advance notice of upcoming events. They should be made to feel like "insiders."

With each subsequent level there are new perks as well as all the attendant perks of the lower gift clubs. The top group, whether it is $1000 or $5000 (the Founders Group or President's Society), might have a distinctive pin or other symbol of identification. These club members should be treated as VIPs and given significant recognition in publications as well as special invitations to events. A special Founders Group luncheon, breakfast, or dinner could be instituted.

It is most likely that in these top two groups of annual fund donors you will discover future major donors. The more effective the cultivation and acknowledgment of their giving, the easier the conversion to a major donor.

The annual fund is the forum for prospecting for new donors. The goal is to double, if possible, or at least to increase their giving each year. This building process helps to develop major donors.

Beyond building and expanding the list, the way in which donors are solicited affects the outcome of the Annual Fund campaign. Donors who have joined the top group deserve a personal visit for solicitation. This indicates to them their value to the organization and greatly enhances the chances of significantly increasing their gift. The organization's resources, both staff and volunteer, determine how many donors can be individually seen and by whom. If the annual fund chairs are willing to visit, include them whenever possible. If they are unable to visit the top group, secure permission to use their name to set up the appointment.

Peer recognition or belonging is a motivator for giving. Ask individuals who have given leadership gifts if their name can be mentioned as a leadership donor when meeting with their colleagues.

The next most effective solicitation method is the personal phone call. Deciding who should call is as important for the outcome as deciding the participants for a personal visit. Again, the annual fund chairs, the dean, or the president might take some names they cannot visit and make the phone call. If it is a school, you can recruit a classmate or two to call some of their class members. If the group is small enough, recruit a committee to canvass their class for annual fund gifts. Calls by students are very effective in generating responses. It is difficult to refuse an enthusiastic student. For nonacademic organizations, a few hand-selected articulate clients can be just as compelling.

No matter where an institution is in the philanthropy process, there should always be an emphasis on the Annual Fund; develop these donors, and development dollars will grow.

CHALLENGE GIFTS

In an annual campaign or capital campaign, a challenge gift can provide a powerful rationale for giving. A challenge gift is a gift of significant size in which a donor agrees to match gifts to the institution by a certain formula. It can be a one-to-one match, which requires $1 in funding to be raised before it is matched dollar-to-dollar by the donor. The equation can be whatever the donor and institution design. It could require a two-to-one match, which necessitates $2 to be raised before it is matched with $1 from the challenge donor.

The donor can put a cap on the maximum to be matched, which controls the cost of their gift. Additionally, the challenge might require that only new gifts would be matched. This is most effective in building your donor base. It provides a compelling reason to approach individuals to become donors.

The donor can set a minimum for giving before their match will begin. For example, the donor could require $50,000 to be raised and only match the additional dollars raised after the $50,000 threshold was met.

The value of a challenge gift is that it can attract new donors and raise the sights of existing donors. Before accepting a challenge gift, determine if the ratio of the match and donor requirements are realistic for the institution. Despite the benefits, there needs to be a level of comfort about the match. If the amount to be raised is too high for the institution to succeed, neither party will be pleased. The background and experience of your donors also needs to be considered. For example, some potential donors respond to "challenges" more than other types of solicitation. Determine whether a challenge gift will motivate donors to increase their giving.

UNRESTRICTED GIFTS

These types of gifts provide the maximum flexibility for the institution. Sometimes donors are so committed to the institution that they do not want to encumber their philanthropy by setting limits or restrictions on their gift. They believe the institution will make the best decision to maximize the impact of their gift. Such gifts are truly prized because they allow the administration the ultimate flexibility to use the gift for a purpose or need that is a priority of the institution. Most annual fund gifts are unrestricted and are used for current operations.

In an academic setting, an attractive option to present to donors is the discretionary gift. The deans and president have discretionary funds that can be used for special projects or priorities that may arise for ongoing or emerging needs. Deans often use these funds to purchase special equipment or to provide resources for faculty or student presentations or attendance at conferences.

No matter the type of gift, restricted or unrestricted, there is an attendant need for recognition and reporting on the gift's use. All donors enjoy being thanked and want assurance that their philanthropy is useful to the institution.

RESTRICTED GIFTS

Restricted donations are, as the name implies, funds given to an institution that are limited or restricted by the donor. The most common restriction is the purpose of the gift. The gift can be designated solely for program support, capital needs, endowment, or scholarship. Within these categories, gifts can be further defined to be used for a specific discipline or department. It can be designated for a building project and, within that context, for a specific area or naming opportunity in the building.

Endowment can be established by donors with very narrow parameters; for example, providing scholarship support for students from a particular city or state, or for children of employees of a particular company.

Restricted gifts should be carefully reviewed by administration and, as appropriate, legal counsel should be sought to ensure that requirements are commensurate with federal and state regulations and consistent with the institution's mission. Occasionally, such gifts are not in the best interest of the institution, and need to be altered to be appropriate, or even refused.

When possible, it is desirable to encourage donors to craft their preferences in such a way that allows for some latitude. This applies especially with endowments that are permanent; much can change within 10, 20, 50 years or more.

Donors want to help the institution and it is incumbent on the institution and its representatives to guide the gift process in such a manner that will fulfill the donor's desires and meet the institutions' needs.

OUTRIGHT GIFTS

Outright gifts are tangible gifts of cash, securities, publicly traded stock, government bonds, municipal bonds, mutual funds, stock warrants, or closely held stock. For cash gifts, individuals are allowed to deduct up to 50% of their adjusted gross income based on the cost of their gift. Gifts of appreciated securities are deductible up to 30% of the donors' adjusted gross income. Highly appreciated securities are good vehicles for gifting, as donors can minimize or avoid capital gains tax, thus reducing the cost of the gift. If used for a life income plan, it allows the donor to convert the stock to a more secured income level without incurring the capital gains tax for appreciation. Appreciated securities are particularly good gift vehicles because the donor receives a charitable tax deduction and escapes capital gains. For example, assuming the stock was purchased for $50/share several years ago but is now worth $100/share, some capital gains tax would be assessed for the $50 increase.

Real estate gifts allow the donor to convert the property through a planned gift to an income-producing asset. Gifts of property and real estate need to be valued by a qualified independent appraiser to establish a fair market value (FMV) for the gift. These gifts should be carefully reviewed by legal counsel. If the property is mortgaged or has some environmental hazards, certain restrictions or considerations should be followed carefully.

Life insurance policies that are no longer useful can provide an attractive tax savings. An individual can purchase a new policy naming the institution as beneficiary and if structured properly premiums could qualify for charitable deductions. This might be an avenue for some younger donors to make a substantial eventual gift to the institution.

There are special restrictions on gifts of artwork. The amount of the deduction is contingent on the nature of the gift and its purpose and the use or sale of the artwork.

The primary motivation for donors is belief in the institution rather than tax incentives for giving. For committed individuals, it can be helpful to demonstrate the real cost of the gift after all possible deductions.

The simplest gift is the outright cash gift. It is immediately applicable to the need and its use is clear.

BEQUESTS

An individual's will documents their final wishes concerning the wealth accumulated over a lifetime. Upon death, the executor distributes the individual's worldly possession to family, friends, and to those institutions that have affected the individual's life in a positive way. This distribution is called a bequest. This is the least complicated type of "planned gift."

A bequest can be established for your institution by a donor with a simple codicil or clause added to an existing will. An attorney on the board can provide samples for your donors to discuss with their advisors. It is very easy for donors to add a codicil or include instructions in their will or revocable living trust that will guide the executor in managing the bequest. The donor should retain legal counsel before making will revisions. Sample wording could be suggested by legal counsel similar to the following: "I give to _____ (institution) ____ (state) a nonprofit corporation located in (city/location) _____(state) ____, the sum of ($100,000) to establish the John and Mary Smith Endowment Fund for the School of Nursing, income to be used for gerontological nursing."

Another option is to transfer property via the will. Possible language would indicate something such as "I give to (institution), a (state) nonprofit corporation located in (city) my personal residence located at (address), (city), (state) to be sold by the (organization) and the proceeds used to establish the (named endowment fund) for (purpose)." It can further stipulate that the income only be used or give permission to invade the principal. In either example, the bequest could simply be a transfer of assets to the institution rather than to endow a fund. An additional option could indicate something similar to "I give (a percentage of) the rest, residue, and remainder of my estate to (nonprofit)." The percentage could be qualified by indicating that it would be the adjusted gross taxable estate and that no reduction is made to the bequest by any state or federal taxes.

An individual can make a bequest to more than one institution or can specify an amount. Also, the individual can specify that the percentage can be limited to a certain amount not to exceed $_____. These examples are offered to give a sense of possible options and language. *Donors should retain legal counsel regarding such gifts.*

A donor can also set up a testamentary trust to pay a relative or other individual or individuals for life or a specified number of years. Upon completion of the terms of the trust, the principal would then become the property of the nonprofit organization.

The benefit to the donor is the tax relief for their estate. This is not an immediate gift to the institution, but an eventual gift. Depending on the terms of the trust and numbers of individuals or percentage of payout or years, the present value of the gift can be affected. For example, a gift of $5,000 in the 1920s was probably a major gift. A gift of $100,000 that is deferred for 20–30 years will not be worth the full $100,000 at the time the gift is actually received. It will be reduced by a certain percentage.

If individuals hold securities, they can authorize what is termed a Transfer on Death or "TOD" to a nonprofit. This shelters these assets from estate tax.

With a bank account or Certificate of Deposit, a Payable on Death or "POD" can be set up in advance. Like the bequest, both of these can include a specified amount or percentage. These instruments insure that the designated funds will go directly to the nonprofit and not through probate, thus avoiding estate taxes.

As stated previously, the bequest is the simplest planned gift for an organization. It is easy to understand and market. If individuals truly value an organization, it is only natural that they will want to see the institution's work continue to perpetuate their own values and beliefs.

It is important to promote bequests with constituents. A simple pamphlet can present the benefits to the institution and legacy for the donor. A special drive could be planned around a significant anniversary for alumni, or it could be included in a capital campaign. Also, solicitation at the time of a special event can yield significant dollars for the future.

There is a certain window of opportunity to encourage bequests. Older donors become reluctant to make changes to their will. They perceive that everything is arranged, and are reluctant to incur the expense and emotion of initiating changes to their will.

Fundraising counting of endowments requires a policy by the board. Some institutions only recognize or count will commitments when they are realized, that is, when the individual dies and the money is received. For some organizations or institutions, the determining factor is the age of the donor. If the individual is in his or her late seventies or eighties, the bequest is counted. Other institutions use some formula that recognizes a portion of the total will commitment.

Will commitments are revocable. Donors can change beneficiaries at will through their will, and sometimes do.

Donors should be encouraged to notify the institution of their bequest. The institution should provide a vehicle and an impetus for the donor to do so. Special attention should be paid to these individuals to let them know how much the institution appreciates this privilege. There are stories of large bequests going to another institution when the initial institution they notified failed to recognize or appreciate an individual's future bequest gift. Most donors have several institutions in their will, so proper recognition can help guarantee remaining in the will. Donors are human, and can vote with their wallets.

FUNDRAISING THROUGH DIRECT-MAIL CAMPAIGNS

Some development activities undoubtedly will be accomplished through direct-mail campaigns. These activities allow contact with a large number of individuals with less time and cost associated with the contact. Direct mail campaigns often entail preparation of a form letter, sometimes with components of the letter targeted to subgroups within the larger group designated to receive the letter. For example, if the letter is going to be sent to all alumni of the school, there might be a separate or different introductory or concluding paragraph for alumni who are celebrating 5, 10, 15, 20, and so on anniversary years since graduation. There may also be a special section of the letter added for previous donors.

To assist with direct mail campaigns, development staff can recruit a board member or prominent volunteer to sign letters. This is especially effective if the volunteer has a relationship with the recipient. In an appeal for reunion gifts, a letter signed by a popular class member could generate increased contributions.

As with other fundraising activities, to the extent possible, a direct mail request should target the potential donor; segment and personalize as much as possible. Accuracy in addressing the request also is extremely important. If a person prefers to use his or her professional credentials, that is, Dr., it is important to use this salutation rather than any other. Many individuals do not like to receive a solicitation letter with an introductory statement that uses their first or familiar name. Do this only if you know the individual well, and if he/she has given you permission to use their first name in salutation or greetings.

Institutions have spent million of dollars in the profit and nonprofit sectors to analyze direct mail results and determine the most successful techniques. Various trends dictated the length and content of the appeal. Some experts espouse that a longer letter, encompassing two to three pages, has greater appeal. The length, they posit, enables the sender to provide more detail to engage the reader and illustrate the need. Others value brevity. There is no magic formula. Most agree that you need to capture your prospect's interest early in the communication to encourage him/her to read the entire message. The length and style should reflect the organization and its constituency.

The content should provide a brief description of the organization, its goals, how long it has been in existence, or some other distinguishing characteristic. The tone should be clear, direct, informative, friendly, and courteous. Consider what method might best illustrate your story. The message could tell the story of a grateful patient recounting the difference that quality health care made in the patient's recovery. This description could encompass an interview using the patient's own words. With this type of presentation, the patient provides the validation of the quality of your educational product. The appeal builds on that premise.

Another frequently used case for support is from the student perspective. Students who receive financial assistance might convey how much this support means in enabling them to pursue their professional education and might include information on future career aspirations.

The case or rationale for support does not have to be a narrative. It could be a straightforward list of services or benefits of the institution and the corresponding needs that support these services.

In a direct-mail solicitation, always ask for a specific amount. If the recipient is a previous donor, past support should be acknowledged and he/she should be thanked for this past support. For example, you could ask these individuals to join a higher level of the gift club or extend an invitation to double last year's gift. The minimum ask should be a request to renew membership in the club or repeat last year's gift. If there are premiums attached to categories of giving, be certain to clearly present these benefits of increased support. For lapsed donors or individuals who have not contributed for 1 to 3 years, a special appeal might rekindle their interest and support. Tell them you have missed their support, and remind them of the value of your organization. Individuals who have never given are the most difficult to convince and often require numerous contacts. Some may resist even the most compelling request. Creativity and patience are required to engage this group.

The text, or an accompanying document or return envelope, should include information on options for giving. If this is a one-time request for annual funds and the preferred contribution is cash, the request should not discuss other options.

Always end the direct-mail letter with information about the time frame of the request. For example, if you are seeking funds before a certain deadline, make that information known to the recipient. Include the name, title, phone number, and email address for the development officer or contact person so that the person can obtain additional information or options for giving.

It may be helpful to prepare a couple samples of the direct-mail appeal and seek input from board members or others close to the institution to enhance appeal and target the message. You might consider sending a sample mailing using two different letters coded to track responses. This obviously requires a longer time frame. Consideration of time frame should be an integral component in the planning process. Allow sufficient lead time and, if at all possible, mail first class. Planning should also estimate the timing when the mail will be received. Avoid the days coinciding with holidays or tax season.

There are consultants and businesses devoted to direct mail marketing. Hiring an expert could help launch or jump-start a direct-mail campaign. Make certain there is a clear understanding of the potential for return and cost incurred to secure each donor prior to hiring a consultant.

Direct-mail solicitations also can be combined with other forms of written communication that you are sending to individuals. For example, any newsletter, alumni magazine, or other form of written communication that may be sent should always include information on how the individual could contribute financial resources to the institution. Different formats can be effective, from an envelope preprinted with the giving options and postage affixed, to an insert inside a magazine.

An emerging avenue for direct-mail campaigning is the Internet. For prospects with e-mail addresses and their permission for contact, you could e-mail the request. If you have a web site, be certain to include information about ongoing needs, current appeals, methods, benefits of giving, and contact person.

Packaging is an integral aspect of the message. No matter how straight-forward the solicitation is, whether a simple letter and envelope or a special brochure with a solicitation enclosed, the package needs to have strong visual appeal. It must be distinctive to increase the chances of being opened and eliciting a positive response. An investment in a well-designed piece can be well worth the cost.

Although direct-mail approaches are probably the most frequently used strategy for much of the fundraising in the United States, they often are most effective when combined with other strategies. They can be excellent supplements to a more personal contact that can be made through phone-a-thons or personal phone calls. The results of direct mailings will increase exponentially with phone calls or personal visits.

FUNDRAISING THROUGH SPECIAL EVENTS

Special events provide unique opportunities to engage in every aspect of the development process. Many activities that are routine for the school or health care institution can evolve into special events that have a development component. In fact, many of the larger schools of nursing and medicine have staff members in the development offices who have primary responsibility for planning, coordinating, implementing, and evaluating special events. Examples of special events can include celebrations recognizing scholarship recipients, award ceremonies for outstanding faculty and staff, donor recognition events, historical celebrations and, of course, alumni activities, especially reunions.

In implementing a comprehensive development program within the school or institution, it is wise to consider every event a "special event" for fundraising purposes. Sometimes, the event will help gather information about the individuals who are prospects; or serve as a forum to publicly thank past donors for their previous contributions; or introduce potential donors to other individuals who have already made a significant gift. A special event also might identify future board members or new candidates for an executive committee. Never underestimate the potential of special events for individual contact, recognition and honoring potential, and an entrée for follow-up meetings or individual solicitation.

It is wise to be as inclusive as possible in inviting individuals to special events. Remember that politics (and development) rely on the art of inclusion. A special event may spark the interest of a particular individual prospect bringing them closer to the institution.

As with all other fundraising activities, the development staff and the dean or executive must prepare for the special event. Development personnel must carefully cull attendance lists so that the dean or executive and the development officer know the background of the individuals attending, including the history of any gifts, previous relationships, and contacts. To ensure attendance, staff should call primary prospects and personally invite them to confirm their attendance. Likewise, ask these individuals to invite and if possible escort new prospects who might be interested in the organization. This will help build your prospect base.

There should be enough staff available to host the key donors or prospects. This will maximize opportunities to advance cultivation. Their role is to become acquainted with the prospect. The staff person initiates the cultivation and begins to develop the relationship. Through this dialogue, they can discuss activities of the organization that might be of particular interest to the prospect. Events provide the backdrop to promote the mission, benefits, or special features of the organization. When appropriate, there should be a display that presents some services or accomplishments. If the event does not lend itself to a display, the printed program or a brochure should include this information. Another option might be a continuous video of the organization's mission and community contribution playing in an adjoining room or on the side of the room.

Follow-up from the special event is as important as the invitation. If an individual expresses interest in more information about a specific program or activity, for example, someone should be assigned the follow-up to make certain the contact is made. A debriefing should follow all special events, to record any information that is relevant to fundraising.

Events can be fundraisers such as the "Nightingala" discussed in chapter 10. The simplest method for a fundraising event is to enlist table sponsors and offer them special perks. The sponsor agrees to a higher price for the table in exchange for some recognition. Often the development staff can solicit companies for sponsorships through their marketing or philanthropic funds. Friends of the organization should also be invited to be sponsors. Recognition as a sponsor could be as minimal as the company name on signage for a dinner banquet, or a listing in the Sponsor category on the program and/or invitation. Sometimes presenting a keepsake or memento at registration or at the place setting is helpful in the fundraising process. These can be specially designed pins, ornaments, or a decorative or accessory item. These mementos should reflect your organization. If well designed, they can serve as a cultivation piece long after the event.

There can be tiers of sponsorship or varying levels of ticket prices; each may have specific incentives for that category. For example, the top sponsors might have a dinner or luncheon at the chief executive's home. If a celebrity guest is the guest of honor or the attraction for the event, the premium for this level of support could be a cocktail party or intimate gathering. Sometimes there are different venues entirely for dinners, ranging from formal to informal. In some cases, organizations have held these events on different evenings. This approach, which can be more lucrative, deserves a cautionary note, as some of your supporters could be offended.

Another tried and true fundraising event is an auction, either silent or with a celebrity auctioneer. An auction usually requires a major time commitment and sophisticated volunteer structure. A committee is assigned to canvass retailers for auction items well in advance of the event. Site selection, publicity, and attractive display of the auction items are other key components.

Before initiating a fundraising event, it is wise to check with other organizations in the area so you are not competing for the same individuals and to avoid conflicts in dates. Sometimes organizations have found it beneficial to join together to host an event, either for public relation purposes or fundraising.

Before engaging in any special fundraising activity or fundraising event, assess staff and volunteer strengths to determine if this is the best use of resources—the cost-to-benefit ratio. Although the benefits of special events to the overall development goals are many, these activities are staff-intensive.

Direct mail and special events are important for developing your donors. Direct mail is the foundation for the Annual Fund campaign. Once the format for the campaign is decided it can be updated annually to increase its effectiveness based on current data and results. Special events increase the visibility of the institution. They also provide a list of names for future solicitations. Together direct-mail campaigns and special events enhance the overall fundraising plan.

DEVELOPMENT OFFICER'S PERSPECTIVE

From a fundraiser's standpoint, any gift is welcome. One is not intrinsically better than another. The challenge for a development officer is to make certain that the money raised is for a purpose central to the institution and that the method of "gifting" is not so encumbered that its usefulness is hindered.

Immediate or outright gifts are always welcomed by the institution. Gifts that have a payout in 5 or 10 years are also very attractive. Conversely, if several family members receive income for their lifetimes, the real value of the eventual gift could be diminished. Endowment gifts are favored over bequests, because bequests are revocable and can be altered to suit the donor's latest wishes. No matter what type of gift is associated with the donor, always remember to "cherish that donor."

Specialized fundraising activities such as direct-mail campaigns and events are components of a comprehensive development plan. All fundraising activities must be continuously evaluated toward the goal of enhancing revenues.

DEAN'S OR EXECUTIVE'S PERSPECTIVES

Before asking any donor for a gift, it is important to be clear about the priorities of the school. If there were an urgent need for scholarship funds for current students, it would make sense to first approach potential donors who have the potential to give outright gifts. In the case of outright gifts, the next step is determining whether the donor would like to have it used now, or would like to have only the interest used, in which case the gift would last for future generations of students. Open, direct, and clear communication with donors and potential donors is one of the most important aspects of the development process. Often, the responsibility for designing the content of the communication lies with the dean. The development officer then backs up the dean in continuing communications with the donors. A team approach ensures success.

5

Reasons for Giving

JOYCE J. FITZPATRICK AND SANDRA S. DELLER

M any things can happen in an individual's life to motivate him or her to engage in gift giving on some level. In fact, caring for others in a community-spirited manner is often taught to young children as they participate in food drives at schools and in church. Although motivation to help others who are less fortunate is often cited as one of the reasons for gift-giving, it is not the only motivating factor.

One of the many challenges of the fundraising process is to figure out what might motivate a prospective donor to make a gift. Often, the goal is to match the needs of the prospective donor with the needs of the institution for funds.

There may be as many reasons why people will give to a particular cause as there are prospective donors. The most important factor to remember is that this individual's reasons for wanting to give his or her own funds are very personal, and at many times, very private. Respect for the individual's motivation for giving is paramount to those who are managing the development process. It also goes without saying that it is important to respect the privacy and confidentiality of the donors and prospective donors, to the extent that they wish their stories to be private.

From the analysis of gift-giving over the years, some themes have been identified in motivations for giving of personal resources. These include:

1. desire to memorialize others, particularly loved ones;
2. desire to leave a personal legacy;
3. interest in recognition;
4. commitment to give something back for the rewards received;

5. interest in perpetuating one's own beliefs;
6. desire to belong;
7. guilt; and
8. affinity to programs and goals of institution.

Each of these themes is discussed below.

Desire to Memorialize Others, Particularly Loved Ones

Many of us feel indebted to family and close personal colleagues for all that they have done to help us be who we are, whether personally or professionally. When it comes time to recognize someone to whom we are indebted, often we chose to memorialize him or her by making a gift in their name. For example, a donor may be indebted to parents for the many sacrifices that they made in order to pay for their college education. Thus, they may choose to name an endowment fund after their parents, and to have the fund used for support of undergraduate students, as a legacy to their parents' support of their undergraduate education. Many individuals find this a very easy way to name a fund, and thus, the gift and the benefits of the gift have a very special meaning for the individual donor.

Throughout our lives, many of us have learned ways to pay honor and respect to loved ones or revered members of our society or families who have died. fundraising provides another avenue for recognizing the gifts of others who have gone before us and have contributed in some meaningful way to our development, whether personal, professional, or societal.

Desire to Leave a Personal Legacy

Some donors want to have their own name associated with a gift to an institution, and thus, to leave a personal legacy. At times, donors need to be encouraged to name funds after themselves. It may be helpful to suggest to professionally successful alumni that having their name attached to a gift would bring in other gifts in that the success of the individual would be associated with the institution. Many of us want to be remembered in perpetuity, and the naming of an endowment fund will provide a personal legacy. This personal naming may be especially important to individuals who do not have children who will carry the family name through the next generations. The recognition of self should not be overlooked with any donor, as it is often the most powerful argument that can be made in favor of a major gift. The majority of potential donors want to leave a personal legacy; naming the gift after themselves is the most direct way to do this.

A donor may achieve both the satisfaction of leaving a personal legacy and recognizing loved ones by naming a gift in the family name, or by combining some family names. The combination of names can be such that they are only interpretable by the donor, or they can be names that are meaningful to others as well. Family named gifts can be designed to accomplish multiple purposes, a recognition of the indebtedness to others as well as a personal legacy. It is not unusual for husbands and wives to wish to honor each other through gifts, by listing the gift in both names.

Interest in Recognition

Just as the individual donor may wish to leave a personal legacy by naming a fund after himself or herself, a gift may also help the individual achieve recognition for their contributions. Donors of major gifts receive recognition in many ways, and for many donors, this recognition is a very important part of the reason for giving. Donors may want this recognition when they retire, on important anniversary dates, for example, the 30-year anniversary of the founding of their company, or on some occasion of celebration at the university or college level. Unless the donor indicates that he or she does not want *any* recognition, it is safe to assume that more is better, and to continue to recognize the donor.

Besides the actual naming of the fund, there are many other ways to give the donor recognition. Honor rolls of donors are most effective, and can take many different forms. It is usual to publish the names of donors and the amount or general level of their gift in annual fund honor rolls, for example. Often, in campaigns for buildings, the donors will be recognized by wall plaques, bricks with their names, or other such symbols. Gift trees are popular among some groups, where each leaf in the tree recognizes a certain level of gift. Almost all alumni publications recognize their donors, in an effort to attract additional donors. The donor and his or her gift can be profiled in a feature story on the life and/or career of the donor. Significant honors and accomplishments are included in these feature stories. Generally, the larger the gift, the more publicity the individual is given.

Commitment to Give Something Back
for the Rewards Received

Independent of the naming of a gift, an individual may be motivated to make a gift because they feel indebted in some way for the riches that they have received in life. In many cases, the individuals are aware that the academic institution, and the faculty who taught them, have been an important part of the professional success that they have achieved. Prestigious institutions rely heavily on this indebtedness factor in developing their fundraising initiatives. This desire to give back to others for one's successes can be related to family as well as institution, and more generally, can be related to society.

Often, in fundraising for health care institutions, there is discussion of the "grateful patient," one who is pleased for the competent and caring professionals responsible for the success of treatments. Patients may view their doctors and nurses very positively for having saved their lives. It is well known that grateful patients make very good donors, and every effort should be made to assess patient satisfaction and to translate this into financial support for future good works of the institution.

Interest in Perpetuating One's Own Beliefs

Giving to a particular cause may provide a donor some assurance that his/her beliefs will be perpetuated. Often a donor can be persuaded to give a gift because the goals of the institution or the goals of the specific project for which funding is being sought are consistent with the donor's beliefs and values. Or the donor may specify how the gift is to be used, in order to perpetuate his/her own beliefs. Any specific designation by the donor of the purpose or use of funds is an effort to communicate the donor's interests, values, or beliefs. For example, a donor might want to make certain that their alma mater excelled in the area of geriatric nursing, because she believes that the care of the elderly is the most pressing problem facing health care professionals. Also, a donor could support a particular educational program in nursing or medicine because of their belief that this is the most important way to educate the future generations of health professionals. Perhaps a businessman or businesswoman wants to prepare the next generation of nurse or physician managers, and thus would be willing to support a program in health care management.

Desire to Belong

There are several ways in which the motivation to belong to a particular group can lead one to become a donor. The most widely used example of this in fundraising is the use of the "honor roll," in which individuals who have made donations are listed, and the list is sent out to all donors and potential donors. Often those who have given look for their names on the list; they want to belong to the "in group" of donors and supporters. List of honor rolls also can be used to encourage donors to increase their gifts; the donor or potential donor may want to be listed with others whom they know who have provided certain levels of support.

Guilt

Some donors give gifts because the are driven by guilt. They may feel guilty for their own success, and the gift helps them to atone for their "sins" or grievances. They may feel undeserving of honors and accomplishments, and may want to recognize the contribution that the institution has made to their success. At times, the donor will describe this guilt as the key motivation to their gift-giving, and at times it will be up to the dean and development officer to understand that there is not a need for an explicit statement regarding the motivation.

Affinity to Programs and Goals of Institution

Just as the donor may give a gift to perpetuate his/her own beliefs, it is also possible for him/her to provide support because the programs and goals of the institution fit with personal or professional goals of the donor. This motivation may be closely related to the motivation to perpetuate one's own beliefs. The more that can be done to describe the programs and goals of a particular institution as related to an individual's own beliefs about the topic, the more likely that the donor will want to make a gift.

Many of the motivations described above lead the donor to want some external recognition of the gift. This can be accomplished in any number of ways, and donor recognition is extremely important. For example, the name(s) of the individual(s) who are being memorialized can be attached to endowment funds, programs, classroom space, or lecture halls. The donor may wish to name an endowment fund in recognition of a particular interest, individual, family, or corporation. The most important thing to remember is that it is the donor's wishes that determine the use of the funds and the manner in which the recognition occurs. Yet, it also is the case that many donors are unsure about whether and how they wish the recognition to occur. The dean and development officer can help the donor to figure out the best match of the recognition plan with their personal needs and motivations for the gift. Again, this means that the more that you can learn about the donor, the better you can help meet his or her needs for both gift-giving and recognition.

DEVELOPMENT OFFICER'S PERSPECTIVE

As a development officer, there is nothing so satisfying as the opportunity to assist a prospect to "turn on" to philanthropy. There truly should be a joy in giving. To achieve this requires sensitivity to the donor's values and an appreciation of their compatibility with an institutional need. When there is a match, it is a marriage of interest and need. The donor may become so enthusiastic about the project that they will stretch to fund the goal required or accelerate pledge payments; some have been known to solicit support for their new project from relatives, friends, or associates. Prospects who have become donors have expressed to me that they feel that they have gotten so much more than they gave.

DEAN'S PERSPECTIVE

Understanding the donor's motivation for giving is as important as any other component of the fundraising process, in particular because it allows you to build a gift-giving scenario with the donor that meets the needs of both the donor and the school. The key to identifying the motivation of the donor is listening to their story about who they are and what motivates their interest in a potential gift. The challenge is to identify the best match between what is motivating the donor and the needs of the school so as to maximize the gift. The more closely the gift matches the donor's needs, the more satisfied they will feel about the entire gift-giving process.

6

Individual Gifts

Joyce J. Fitzpatrick and Sandra S. Deller

Individual gifts represent the largest source of private funding. In 1998, according to the data available from GIVING USA, personal giving by living individuals represented the vast majority of charitable contributions, 77.3%, totaling $134.84 billion, nearly a 10% increase over the 1997 number. Giving by individuals has increased significantly for 3 consecutive years, from 1996 through 1998. Also, relatedly, bequest giving continues to rise, by approximately 7.8% in 1998 to reach $13.62 billion (AAFRC Press Release, 1999).

Given this information, and the potential for increasing individual gifts, it makes sense that much of the fundraising activity should be concentrated in this area. Yet, because individual gift-giving is just that—individual—it takes more time and concentrated energy to build the relationship and to implement a solicitation and stewardship process. Once the decision is made about the number of major gifts that are sought for a particular fundraising goal or program, the next decision should be: What percentage of these gifts can be expected from individual donors? Certainly, individual gifts should be expected to account for more than half of any campaign goal, and should be targeted as contributing somewhere between 50–90% of the overall goal. These individual gifts may be of many different types, for example, cash, outright gifts of stock or property, planned gifts, including annuities or insurance policies, and will commitments and bequests.

Consider the following two gifts as examples of major individual gifts. Oseola McCarty was a washerwoman who became known throughout the United States when she gave away her life savings of $150,000 to help

44

complete strangers get a college education at the University of Southern Mississippi in her home town. According to the *New York Times* obituary, published on September 28, 1999, a day after her death, Miss McCarty had not even known exactly what the word "philanthropy" meant when she decided to give her money to the university. In anticipation of her death, in the summer of 1995, at the age of 89, McCarty decided to give away her savings, representing practically all the money she had ever earned, so that children would not have to work as hard as she did. As a result of her gift and the publicity surrounding it, more than 600 donors added some $330,000 to the scholarship fund. McCarty was a humble woman who did not want any monuments or proclamations regarding her gift, yet she grew to enjoy the attention and notoriety that her gift brought to her. After learning of her gift, Ted Turner, a multibillionaire, was reported to have said: "If that little woman can give away everything she has, than I can give a billion." Turner then proceeded to give away a billion dollars.

Consider the recent gifts of multibillionaire Bill Gates, reputed to be the wealthiest person on the planet, who committed $1 billion in funds to minority scholarships throughout the country. The $17 billion foundation that he set up, the Bill and Melinda Gates Foundation, is focused on education and global health. An inversion of the usual rules for family foundations, it is Bill Gates' father, William H. Gates, Jr., who heads the foundation. The Gates Foundation is the largest in the country, surpassing the second-place David and Lucile Packard Foundation by more than $3 billion and the third-place Ford Foundation by $6 billion. Some of the projects supported recently through the Gates Foundation include $100 million to reduce delays in the delivery of new vaccines to children around the world, $50 million to the Maternal Mortality Reduction program at Columbia University, $50 million for research on the malaria vaccine, and $25 million to the AIDS vaccine initiative. The Foundation also has given about $200 million to the library project, responsible for installing computers and Internet connections in 1,745 libraries in 32 states.

Are there similarities between these two gifts, even though the size of the gifts differs significantly? First, the personal involvement of the individuals is important. Both donors have gifts named after themselves. Second, the donors have committed personal funds to areas that are important to them. Each has chosen the specific focus of the gift. And, third, each has appreciated the publicity surrounding their gift, even though they may not have directly sought out the publicity.

Fundraisers often speak of friend-raising as the first stage of fundraising. In seeking individual gifts, friend-raising is the most important aspect of the process, as the development of a relationship with a potential donor is significant in the overall success of the fundraising initiative. The level of the relationship may indeed determine the nature and amount of the gift. For people give to people more frequently that they give to projects per se.

What are the steps in individual friend-raising and individual fundraising? Consider the following as key components: (a) identification of key individuals as prospects for gifts; (b) building of the relationship; (c) research and maintenance of the records; and (d) nurturing the relationship over time, involvement and stewardship of the individual. Each of these aspects will be discussed in some detail, with specific examples given to illustrate the key points. Both the executive and the development officer should be involved in all phases of fundraising for individual gifts. In fact, it helps to have someone else to work with so that, through the team approach, you can maximize your efforts. For example, if the executive has a close relationship with the potential donor because of his or her positional leadership role, the development officer can make certain that the conversation stays focused toward gift potential, and that casual conversation is directed toward obtaining information about the potential donor and his/her interests, financial resources and commitments, family obligations, other philanthropic projects, and financial plans for the future. If the development officer has the stronger relationship due to common interests, for example, the executive can make certain the conversation remains focused on the goals of the fundraising. In all cases, it is important for the executive and the development officer to have discussed the strategy for each potential donor prior to any conversations and/or meetings with the prospect.

Identification of Key Individuals As Prospects for Gifts

Every possible source of potential donors should be explored. For a health science school, this could include current students (who will be future alumni); parents, grandparents, relatives, spouses, significant others, and friends of current students; alumni and their parents, grandparents, children, other relatives, spouses, and significant others; and friends of alumni. For both health science schools and health care institutions, potential donors would include any board members or advisory board members;

committee members, staff, including faculty and retired staff and faculty; grateful patients; and individuals who in any way have benefited from the services of the school or institution.

In addition, it is important to remember that past donors are the best future donors. Thus, those who have contributed to previous campaigns should be put on a list of prospects. And individuals who have contributed either large amounts, or have contributed consistently over a period of years, to annual fund drives also should be placed on the list of prospects. The development officer should identify the list of prospects from past records and make these persons known to the executive.

Building the Relationship

Although the nature of the relationship will vary somewhat with each individual prospect and the development team (executive and development officer), there are three important phases: the cultivation phase, the solicitation phase, and the stewardship phase. The time that it takes to progress through each of these phases also will vary, but the goal should always be to move to the solicitation phase as soon as possible.

The cultivation phase of the relationship begins as soon as the individual is identified as a prospect. If the individual is a potential major donor as defined by the institution's history and goals, the first meeting should include the executive. Major donors in large institutions may be those who have potential for gifts over $100,000, while in institutions with no history of fundraising and no donor base, the major gift may be a very modest $1000. The goal is often to get a commitment for as large a gift as possible and build on it for the future. For example, major gift donors for a new campaign often are obtained by reviewing the $1000 donor list from previous annual fund drives.

Orientation of prospects to the strategic plans, goals, and projects of the school or institution should be a key component of the cultivation phase of the relationship. Efforts should be directed toward ascertaining the potential donor's interests that might be a match with the goals of the school or institution. The presentation of the materials and the communication with the prospective donor should be as clear and direct as possible. Communication should be succinct and honest, and of course, responsive to the prospect's questions and concerns. It is important, however, to remember that making the case for need is not sufficient; donors want to support institutions where there also is vision combined with need.

The cultivation phase may include a wide array of activities that are oriented to getting the individual acquainted with the institution. Often, the introductory phase consists of a breakfast, lunch, or dinner meeting; of course, the choice of meal is centered around the potential donor's schedule, interest, and convenience. At any meeting that is scheduled it is helpful to have both team members present, i.e., the executive and the development officer, so that they can assist each other in keeping the conversation focused and flowing. At the same time, they can pick up and mentally record different cues from the prospect. In scheduling any meeting with a potential donor, it is important to let them know who will be attending, and what the purpose of the meeting will be. It also is important to determine whether or not the individual will be accompanied by anyone else. If the potential donor's spouse will be key to the decision regarding the gift, it may be wise to invite him or her to the introductory meeting.

In the cultivation phase of a relationship remember that contrary to the general belief, most people do like to talk about themselves. To the extent possible, it is important to listen to the individual's story, to draw them out as much as possible, and to gather as much information about them as will be useful to the development process.

Building the relationship with prospective donors implies a direct personal contact. Major gifts are not usually obtained through phone calls, letters, or indirect forms of communication. Most people want a personal relationship with their philanthropy; they may want the "high touch" approach that is so characteristic of the helping professions such as nursing. Donors generally want to be involved in the institution; they want to know what is going to happen to their contribution.

It goes without saying that interpersonal skills are the cornerstone of fundraising with individuals. Communication skills are key to good interpersonal relationships. However, knowledge and understanding of the culture of the individual and the society in which they live are equally important aspects of the interpersonal relationship. Fundraising involves an openness to those of different cultures, from different backgrounds, and often with very different beliefs. The executive and development officer must have an accepting and open attitude about those from different cultures. Often, the donor may feel a need to "lecture" you about their beliefs and attitudes. It is important to listen and to understand their background in the context of the institution that is seeking support.

One of our mentors in the fundraising community, an individual who helped raise many millions for a large medical school, suggested to us that in looking for major donors we should always look for the eccentric personalities. His belief was that the eccentrics often were more interested in the recognition and the "audience" that a major gift to an institution would assure. When considering the two major donors mentioned in the beginning of this chapter, it is easy to see how either could be described as "eccentric": Gates, the college dropout, and McCarty, the washerwoman. Many other examples of individuals who are eccentric and have made surprise gifts to worthy causes, usually through bequests, are cited daily in the newspapers. On the other hand, eccentricity is not enough; it would not be wise to look for major donors among all college dropouts.

In the process of fundraising with individual donors, the executive and development officer should involve other individuals who could assist in the cultivation phase. Individuals often give to peers; therefore, if there is someone who is in the same social circle who could assist you in the cultivation process, do not hesitate to engage them. However, before engaging a third party in the process, it is important to be very clear with the third party what the goal is. It is also important that the third party understands and values the goal. It is most helpful if the third party is not only a peer or the prospect, but also a major donor to the institution.

The second phase of the relationship is the solicitation phase. The amount of time for this phase varies, often based on the length of the relationship with the prospect and their previous involvement with the institution. While solicitation is covered separately in another chapter of this book, the key principles of solicitation for individual donors are important to highlight here as well. These include the following:

1. Develop a clear plan; know what the goal of the solicitation with this particular prospect is; determine the possible nature and level of the gift before meeting with the individual for the solicitation.

2. Understand as much about the prospect as possible before going into the solicitation phase and meeting; gain information about their interests, projects, culture, frame of reference, and so on, in order to target your request to match their potential interest in a gift.

3. Maintain communication in an information-seeking mode; ask open-ended questions whenever possible; and be certain that there is a planned solicitation strategy. The executive and development officer should have predetermined, for example, who will ask for the gift. Often, a role-playing or rehearsal of the solicitation plan is in order, especially if the prospect is new to the institution, or if the executive and development officer have not worked together for a long period of time.

4. Always monitor both verbal and nonverbal communication. Prospects may tell you as much by their nonverbal behavior as they do with their verbal behavior.

5. Have an exit plan, so that both the executive and development officer know what possible next steps will be taken. Before the solicitation meeting, the executive and development officer should have discussed alternatives, contingencies, and future strategies. There should be no surprises in the communication between executive and development officer; both should fully understand the plan for solicitation of the prospect.

Throughout the solicitation phase, remember that it is the donor who designates the nature and purpose of the gift. If they truly do not care what the focus of the gift is because of a deep commitment to the institution, it is still wise to share your choice of gift destination with the donor, and make certain that they understand all aspects of how the gift will be used and publicized. Even if they do not want to determine the use of the gift, they may want to determine how the gift will be publicized. Not many donors want to remain anonymous; if they have reasons why they want to remain anonymous, their wishes must be respected. If they are uncertain what the value of the publicity would be, you can share with them the story of the McCarty gift, a gift that led to others, and increased overall donations substantially.

The third phase of the relationship is that of stewardship. With the understanding that a happy donor has potential for future donations, every effort should be made to continue a positive relationship with donors. They should be involved to the extent that they are interested. They should be invited to all major activities; it is then their choice to say no. No one likes to feel as if they are on the outside; therefore, when in doubt, be inclusive.

No executive should go into a solicitation meeting without a brief report on the prospect. In other words, they should be briefed on the individual. This briefing should be confidential and in writing, prepared by the development officer based on all of the information that is available to date. It should include names of the donor(s), including preferred names such as nicknames, salutations, and so on; personal history; giving history to this institution, and to others if large and related in purpose; and suggested "ask," that is, amount and nature of the gift that should be requested based on prospect rating. If the executive is attending a reception or luncheon or dinner with many major prospects, this information should be available on each potential major donor.

Research and Maintenance of the Records

Accurate and comprehensive records are key to successful fundraising. A system should be put in place for all individuals who are involved in all phases of the fundraising process, so that records are complete. These records should include the time and date of each contact with the prospect; the nature of the contact; who participated in the contact; the content of the communication; the outcomes; and the recorder of the information. A solicitation strategy is a key component; this is simply a statement of the rationale for support and the dollar goal, the timeline, if known, and any solicitors identified. No information should be dismissed, as there is no substitute for information obtained directly from the prospect.

Research in various databases can lead to a large amount of information on each of us, especially now in the information age, when much is available for the asking through the Internet. Research is key to understanding the individual; careful interpretation of the data is paramount. To the extent possible, information obtained via secondary sources should be verified, indirectly, of course, in conversations with the prospect. Further, it is very possible for errors to be perpetuated in databases that are copied one to another, so if there is a key piece of information it is best to verify it with the prospect.

Not all information is equal. The development team may have to sort and sift through a great deal of information in order to synthesize it and relate it to the fundraising goals of their institution. Information-gathering for its own sake costs money. Only when the information is put to use in fundraising can it make money. Further, information can help to determine the right solicitor—another aspect of the strategic plan for solicitation.

Throughout the development process, the development officer should be responsible for keeping the database up to date. In particular, it is important to maintain a list of potential major donor prospects, and to remain focused on activities with these prospects. This list should be reviewed periodically for progress that has been made in moving the prospect to a major donor. The more structured the process for review, the more likely that the database will be useful in the fundraising process.

Nurturing the Relationship Over Time

Until the prospect becomes a donor, the relationship must be nurtured over time. Once the prospect becomes a donor, the relationship must again be nurtured over time, so that the donor becomes a future donor. Also, major donors often can lead you to other major donors; if they are believers in the institution, they can "tell the story" more convincingly. Once prospects become donors, involve them in the public relations activities of the fundraising campaign or initiative.

DEVELOPMENT OFFICER'S PERSPECTIVE

Individual fundraising requires approaching each prospect with an open mind, armed with all the data the institution and its resources can supply. There is a strategic plan for targeting the moves, but the plan needs to be dynamic, similar to looking through binoculars to achieve the perfect focus. Even if the individual has been known to the institution for a long time, do not assume that he or she has not grown or that their interests have been refined or changed. Perhaps an event in their lives has made a major impact, and as a result, they have a new commitment. Keep this in mind with regard to your institutional priorities. Inform them of new directions and they just may decide to invest again.

We discussed chemistry in the context of the dean and development officer. This elusive factor also enters into individual fundraising. The development officer must be honest in assessing if he or she is the appropriate individual to develop the relationship. If not, the professional needs to be proactive in enlisting someone else if necessary. Too often, there is a tendency to persist, and the process is stalled. This also can occur with the relationship with the dean. Personalities are just that, personal, and we cannot change them easily, so we need to respect them and adapt.

Check the facts reported in the records. In my many years in fundraising I have discovered husbands and wives who were reported deceased greet me at the house or answer phones when I called for an appointment. The date of graduation recorded is not always correct, or identification with a class may vary due to interrupted education.

While individual giving is on the rise, a recent article in The Chronicle of Philanthropy stated in a recent article, on October 21, 1999: "While the total dollar amount of giving has been increasing, for three decades Americans have never given more than 2.1 per cent of their annual pre-tax income to charity. Not only that, but giving by individuals has not exceeded 1.6 per cent of gross domestic product, which measures the nation's output of goods and services (Billitteri, 1999, p. 1)." In summary, the Chronicle characterized charitable giving as "stuck in neutral."

Value the individual in your prospect pool by being selective in the attention and communication they receive and the method preferred: calls, mail, fax or e-mail. In this era of e-commerce and impersonal communication, making calls and interacting face-to-face with prospects is still the key to major gifts. People give to people. This fundraising mantra remains true.

DEAN'S PERSPECTIVE

Relationships are everything in fundraising with individuals, cherish them and they will reap rewards. Sometimes the rewards will be in direct funds committed to the institution. At other times the prospect may lead you to other potential donors. In this way, one of the goals should be to build a network of individuals who can be beneficial to your institution.

Also, keep in mind the fact that relationships that are developed in the course of fundraising for your institution will last forever. Some will turn into professional relationships; some will even turn into friendships. Never be surprised about the power of the personal connection with another individual around a mutual goal.

SUMMARY

In summary, individual solicitation is key to any fundraising activity. As the plan for development is unfolded, it might be wise to keep the following questions in mind:

1. Given the increase in the number of Americans with annual incomes above $1 million, how many are on your board?
2. How many of these individuals are among your constituents?
3. Do you know how to find the ones who are among your constituents?
4. Who among your staff, board, and volunteers knows these individuals and would be prepared to ask them for a gift?
5. To what purpose would you direct their gift within the strategic plan of your organization?
6. Would you contribute $1 million to the organization that you represent?

REFERENCES

AAFRC Press Release. (1999, May 25). *Total giving increased 10.7% in 1997.* http://www.aafrc.org

Billitteri, T. J. (1999). Moving giving off the dime. *Chronicle of Philanthropy, 12,* 1–2.

7

Planned Giving

Duncan Hartley

Twenty-five years ago, planned giving flourished in the small liberal arts colleges and a few of the Ivy League universities throughout the nation. In many of the smaller colleges, planned giving became a sophisticated and tremendously successful way to raise major funds for endowment and other special purposes. Planned giving officers often had a reporting relationship to the president of the institutions, as many still do, and in some cases becoming a planned giving officer was the beginning of a career that eventually led to a college presidency.

Planned giving is such an integral part of major gifts that every major gift officer should have at least a working knowledge of the methods and vehicles of planned giving. A large percentage, if not a majority, of the multimillion dollar gifts that are made to philanthropies are truly planned gifts, or involve a planned giving component. For example, a $10 million gift from an individual to your institution may involve a combination of distributions of cash or appreciated securities over a period of years, a pledge payment that might consist of real estate or commercial property (a gas station was one such property that became part of a gift), a charitable remainder trust, and perhaps the balance in the form of a bequest. Complex gifts of this nature, as all experienced major gift officers know, are very common. In my experience, it is very rare to receive a $10 million check from an individual donor. Wealthy individuals have always realized that large contributions should be made in a way that takes advantage of the nature of their assets and their tax consequences. Almost by instinct, wealthy individual donors are thinking "planned gifts" as they consider major gift commitments to their favorite philanthropies.

For some reason, the famous philanthropies in New York, Washington, DC, and other major eastern cities somehow overlooked the tremendous potential of planned giving. If some of these institutions had a program, it was usually run in the "back office" by someone who handled legal correspondence, and had no special expertise in marketing or major gifts. A few philanthropies took the step of hiring an attorney, or in some cases a staff of attorneys, to promote planned giving. In these larger institutions, the common practice was for planned giving to remain a highly compartmentalized and specialized office within the larger development department. There was very little integration of planned giving into the mainstream of philanthropic fundraising, and the true potential of planned giving was not fully recognized. Nonetheless, some individual planned giving directors became nationally recognized for their ability, and more and more institutions in New York as well as elsewhere became aware that planned giving was worthy of support as a major institutional priority.

A job description of a successful planned giving officer is almost identical with that of a major gift officer. The individual must be able to represent the institution at its best, and to inspire trust and confidence on the part of donors. Professionalism and high ethical standards, along with an authentic interest in meeting others and building relationships with individuals over long periods of time, is absolutely essential. To be successful, the planned giving officer must be as adept at closing gifts as the major gift officer. In addition to these qualities, the planned giving officer must also be able to relate well to attorneys and trust officers, as well as financial planners, and have a real talent for marketing planned giving programs. The most successful individuals in planned giving not only have an innate instinct for those donors who are capable and interested in making large commitments, but also have an encompassing and creative imagination that serves to develop ways to market the idea of planned giving to broad constituencies, many of whom have no known interest in planned giving. The planned giving professional must also have an excellent working knowledge of the planned giving vehicles, the appropriateness of different approaches, and a working knowledge of the basics of estate planning.

The technicalities of planned giving can virtually open the door to philanthropy for many individuals, and it can be very exciting to see the awareness of this potential develop in an individual who deeply desires to do something significant with their accumulated assets. Meeting with a donor who realizes that it is possible to create a professorship, endow a scholarship fund, or perhaps even to provide capital funds for construction through a planned gift is a very moving experience.

A key part of marketing planned giving is educational, but all of the skills of cultivation, follow-up, personal attention, involvement, and asking for the gift are obvious steps. The Moves Management approach to donor cultivation and solicitation, made so popular by Dave Dunlop, formerly of Cornell University, and others, is as effective in planned giving as it is in major gifts. In fact, Dave Dunlop's concept of the Ultimate Gift as the culmination of steps in Moves Management is probably more commonly than not a planned giving commitment (Dunlop, 1986).

Planned giving is essential to a well-balanced and mature development program for most philanthropies. In considering ways in which you can increase the effectiveness of your program, and secure more long-term commitments to support the future of your organization, planned giving is an important aspect of your development program. For colleges and universities, cancer research institutions, and many other major American philanthropies, the planned giving program often is essential. An increased commitment of resources and professional staff, and an awareness of the importance of marketing and the expertise to develop a marketing program, are the necessary elements.

If your organization, however, does not have a long history of planned giving, or executives are uncertain of how successful a planned giving program would be, there may be great hesitancy among chief executive officers and deans as well as other organizational leaders to launch a planned giving program. Often, they are skeptical because they have heard that the results of planned giving may not appear for many years. With nonprofit executives as with corporate executives, there is intense pressure to achieve results now, and very few executives of any kind are interested in enhancing the reputations of the next generation of leaders.

However, two questions should be explored: (1) Will planned giving work for my organization? and (2) How successful will a planned giving program be—how long will we have to wait for the rewards? It is tempting to say that any organization that plans to have a future should have a strong and vital planned giving program. However, some organizations may not be capable of developing an effective program. Small community-based organizations, especially new ones, should probably not make the attempt to invest in planned giving. Any organization that depends upon annual contributions and foundation grants to exist from month to month and year to year probably cannot support an organized program.

In many cases, there is the opportunity to approach a board member or community leader to consider a major planned gift to help assure the future of the organization. There have always been enlightened donors who have done such a thing for small organizations that have not yet achieved wide recognition.

There is another kind of organization that often finds difficulty in developing a professional planned giving program. Some philanthropies receive almost all of their funds from a single source, such as corporate support. An organization that is identified in the minds of its constituencies with a particular source of support may find it extremely difficult to pursue planned giving aggressively. We all know of the executive director of a small organization with insufficient financing that dreams of having an endowment that will permanently support that organization for years to come. This is almost always an unsatisfied dream. As a rule of thumb, the longer the organization has been in existence, and the wider its reputation and constituency, the more likely it is to benefit from planned giving.

The overall success of a planned giving program is usually easy to grasp, but can be somewhat difficult to quantify. In a mature program, between 25% and 30% of the organization's total philanthropic cash income should come through planned giving. Here I am referring to cash income from planned gifts only. This would include income from bequests and charitable trusts that is distributed from estates through executors, and other sources of planned giving cash income. Some consultants feel that if the planned giving income is greater than 30% of the organization's total philanthropic income, then there are weaknesses in other parts of the fundraising program that need to be corrected. However, only the most experienced and professional planned giving programs have already reached this level of philanthropic income generation.

Some organizations are guilty of not counting or crediting a major part of planned giving success. For example, some major organizations only count an irrevocable charitable trust after the death of the last income beneficiary and the distribution of the trust assets to the philanthropy. Very successful planned giving officers who close many trusts a year are given little or no credit for their efforts, and the organization, its board and leadership, are not well informed about the successful activity in the planned giving program. A far better approach is to give credit for the gift when a charitable trust is created. Some organizations give credit at the full fair-market value of the trust at the time of its creation, while other organizations discount this value because the funds will not actually be received by the philanthropy for an uncertain period of time. Counting the gift when it is made is vital to the morale and motivation of planned giving officers and deans and executives, and it also establishes a more visible level of accountability in the planned giving program. How can any philanthropy know how well it is doing if all of its board members and administrators do not know how much money is secured through the planned giving program on an annual basis? It seems simply old-fashioned and a bit reactionary for an organization to exclude such gifts from its annual philanthropic attainment.

There are some other critical measures of a successful planned giving program. Many organizations like to publicize the number of bequest expectancies that they have in their records. Large universities and other philanthropies ordinarily have at least 1,000 bequest expectancies at any given time. Having such a large number of people include you in their wills through a bequest is an indication of the credibility and stature of an organization. This number should grow every year, and it is an extremely important indicator of successful planned giving activity. Of course, as suggested above, the number and value of charitable trusts and similar instruments that are actually established to benefit your organization every year is another indication of results. The number of trusts, and the total value of trusts created, can be reported and compared with previous years. Other important criteria include the number of major planned giving donors under cultivation by staff, and the steps that have been taken to move these donors toward making a gift. The effectiveness of a marketing program can also be gauged by the number of planned giving inquiries that are received and managed by the planned giving staff during the course of a year. In planned giving as in major gifts, the dollars received during a 12-month period do not tell the whole story. Intelligent managers should take all of the above measures into consideration when evaluating the success of a planned giving program.

It also is important to understand that many of the major gifts announced prominently in the national media are often in reality either planned gifts or complex gifts that include a planned giving component. A pledge to a capital campaign of several million dollars over a few years may be "guaranteed" by a bequest to take into consideration that the donor may not live to see the completion of the commitment. Individuals who make very large philanthropic gifts are usually quite aware of the disposition of their assets, and the tax consequences of their giving. They will structure their gifts in ways that best serve their personal circumstances and the needs of the philanthropy. Very often, this will necessarily involve elements of planned giving. In a larger sense, planned gifts and major gifts are inseparably tied through the gift planning process.

FIRST STEPS IN ESTABLISHING
A PLANNED GIVING PROGRAM

Organizations new to planned giving often believe that they have to have (a) a staff member trained in the complexities of charitable life-income trusts; (b) a planned giving committee; and (c) an expensive brochure before they can begin any substantial planned giving as a philanthropic activity. Careful evaluation of staff resources is critical before launching a planned giving program.

A simple approach is usually much more effective, and can actually provide information about what directions to take in building a planned giving program. When these initiatives are taken by an inexperienced organization, the foundation for successful planned giving in the future can be almost hopelessly damaged. The wrong people doing the wrong things at the wrong time with the wrong prospects is the worst possible result. Of course, a staff member does need to be given the responsibility for promoting a planned giving program. When this is a part-time responsibility, there is the danger that the press of everyday events will prevent planned giving from ever really happening. Nonetheless, a first step must be taken by assigning responsibility to a staff member. You will need a one-page explanation of how to make a bequest to your organization with some sample language of how to word a bequest and the suggestion that the prospect consult his/her financial and legal advisors. Include the legal name of your organization and its current address. It is important for an attorney to look at this simple document *before* you start distributing it. You are now in the planned giving business.

One of the most successful small planned giving programs that I heard about years ago was a youth organization on the Main Line in Philadelphia. A very experienced board member who was totally committed to the organization joined with a senior staff member in talking to other loyal constituents of the organization about making planned gifts. It did not take long for several million dollars to be committed. Outstanding volunteer leadership, the mission of the organization, and the loyalty of the organization's constituency were the factors that led to this success. The key thing here is that someone important decided to ask others to make planned gifts. Without this "asking," there would have been no program and no results. This really does not sound very complicated, and it has served as a reminder to me of what the true basics are in planned giving as well as in all of philanthropy.

It is when you decide to go from the basic level of planned giving to a more advanced level that many important questions arise. Should you have a consultant? Should you have a full-time staff member who is highly trained in all of the techniques of planned giving? What about newsletters, advisory committees, and other elements of the complete planned giving package? The simple answer is that you should do some of everything, and continue doing whatever works. Obviously, good judgment and experience become more and more important as you progress along this path.

A survey was recently completed among leading institutions of higher education in this country. The results are extremely interesting, because they show clearly that the cultivation of planned giving prospects is rated the most highly of any activity, while planned giving advisory committees and special events for attorneys and trust officers are both rated extremely poorly. Also highly rated are special events and educational materials for donors, and the ever-neglected stewardship activities for planned giving donors. Ads and stories in university publications received high grades as well. This collective wisdom of major universities is valuable advice for a planned giving practitioner at any level of experience. Obviously, we all want to focus our efforts on what will produce the best results in an economical way during a reasonable period of time. What works best at leading universities will probably work best for your organization as well. Although this survey does not provide a template that you can simply adopt wholesale, it does include a summary of insights and perspectives that can give guidance.

THE PHILANTHROPIC LIFESTYLE

A face-to-face meeting between an experienced planned giving officer and an appropriate prospect is the necessary and essential step that must be taken over and over again in any planned giving program. During the first meeting with a planned giving prospect, you should be able to evaluate the commitment of the individual to your organization, and identify any conflicts or hindrances that may exist between the individual and the desire of that person to support your organization. If there are problems, you may be able to begin discussing them, or at least be able to take them into account in future interactions with this person. You also may be able to gauge the philanthropic intent and the financial resources of the individual, although this is very often much more complicated than it might appear to be. Many extremely wealthy people lead relatively modest lifestyles, drive ordinary cars, take ordinary vacations, and do not flaunt their wealth.

In fact, a landmark study conducted by anthropologists at Yale University interviewing major gift donors to American institutions of higher education identified what they called the "philanthropic lifestyle" that is common to most major gift donors. These individuals have a personal philosophy that the holding of wealth is a privilege, and that it is their responsibility to steward this wealth and to make select gifts to a few philanthropies that will benefit the causes that they believe are most important to the community (Odendahl, 1987). It has been confirmed many times in my experience that people who share these values are indeed the most likely to make truly significant gifts that will support the future of your organization.

The first meeting with a potential planned giving donor is also the beginning of a professional friendship that should exist over a period of years. You should leave every meeting with a clear idea of what the next step will be in this new relationship. Should you see this person again in the near future, or perhaps in a year, or is this someone who should be seen every 2 years? If the individual does not seem to have the strong interest and is not ready to consider a gift now, is it worthwhile to continue cultivating this person by mail? On the other hand, if a strong interest is discovered, and the donor seems to be motivated to act in the near future, should other individuals, such as a president, a dean, or a board member, be involved? In my experience, donors considering gifts of $1 million or more usually want to meet the chief executive officer or some person of similar rank before actually completing the gift. I know of one recent case in which a person committed to a gift with the understanding that he would be introduced to a key volunteer in person. This makes perfect sense because a truly major gift will affect the character and future direction of an organization, at least in some specific way.

MARKETING YOUR PLANNED GIVING PROGRAM

Marketing your planned giving program offers the opportunity for endless innovation. The idea of planned giving, and the benefits that may be enjoyed by the donor and the organization, should be communicated as broadly and as frequently as possible to all of the donors and friends of your organization. This is the ideal meeting place for "high tech and high touch" in fundraising and philanthropy. All of your skills with a fountain pen, a Palm Pilot, and the most complex computer programs can be brought to bear. A significant objective of your efforts should be to get individuals within your constituency to identify themselves as being interested in making a planned gift to support the future of your organization. Frequently, spouses may respond at different times to different kinds of initiatives. As time passes, a friend of your organization will go through the inevitable life changes that involve all of us in one way or another. Because there is no way of predicting when these changes will occur, it is a good strategy to have a continuous flow of initiatives that will inform a person at a time when that individual wishes to have the knowledge that you are providing. This will encourage an important response that will satisfy both the donor and the interests of your organization. Occasional or random mailings or other initiatives are much less effective because they fail to carry on an educational program over time, and they also miss the windows of opportunity that will be occurring in your constituency.

A planned giving newsletter that comes out three or four times a year can be a very effective way to educate people about the benefits of planned giving and encourage them to respond by asking for additional information, or informing you about a gift that they have already made or are contemplating. Newsletters should never be slick and commercial-looking, but they should be serious and well-done. You can safely assume that many of your best prospects are already receiving such newsletters from other organizations, so it is important that your publication be distinctive, and that it reflect clearly the mission and purpose of your organization in a way that invites an emotional commitment. How many newsletters should you send? First of all, it is important for staff to personally handle every response received as a result of your newsletter mailing. It is usually best for one person to have the responsibility for making all of the appropriate follow-up calls. Other staff members can be involved in visiting the donors or in actually handling the paperwork related to gift-giving.

If you send 10,000 newsletters with a 2% response, you will possibly have 200 responses that must be personally managed by telephone and letter. When you do newsletter mailings, certain questions need to be addressed. Should the response device card be a tear-off postcard, or should it be something that goes inside an envelope marked "confidential"? Should the response device simply ask for a person's name and telephone number, and offer a check box or two for more information? By giving the person an option to write in their telephone number and the best times of day to call, you can increase the quality of your responses, but the percentage of overall response will probably drop. You also want to have donors feel free to write comments on the card. A donor who sends in a card with handwritten comments is much more likely to be a prospect than one who does not. Perhaps there should be a section at the bottom asking for comments. As in direct mail, every change that you make on the card and the newsletter will make a difference in the percentage of response and in the quality of response. Since these may not go hand in hand, you need to evaluate the results very carefully, and continue to refine your mailings.

Warning: Never send out a newsletter unless you are fully prepared to follow up on all of the responses that are received. Nothing is worse than to encourage a donor to express an interest in planned giving, and then to make no response.

There are other extremely effective ways to encourage interest in planned giving. You could consider placing an insert page on planned giving in every issue if your organization's magazine or major publication. This page would include a coupon that could be cut out and returned to you indicating an interest in planned giving. Either an insert page or a full-page bound into the magazine, preferably the inside back cover, can become key elements in your marketing plan. A check-off box on the response device of every direct mail letter is a good idea, and has been tested by some organizations to make sure that it does not interfere with annual giving results. It does not. There is no good reason not to have a planned giving check-off box in virtually every fundraising mailing. Of course, there is nothing more effective than well-written articles on individuals who have made planned gifts, along with photographs of the donors.

RECOGNIZING PLANNED GIFT DONORS

Donors of every planned gift, including bequest expectancies, should receive prompt and appropriate recognition, including a letter of thanks from the chief executive officer of your organization. Membership in a special planned giving society, listing in donor giving reports, plaques, and special naming opportunities should all be available as means of showing warm appreciation for the generosity of planned giving donors. Unfortunately, this is very often an area of confusion in some organizations. When the gift will not be completed for many years, some organizations feel that immediate recognition is not needed, or perhaps might even be inappropriate. However, a commitment, including a bequest expectancy which is revocable, is nonetheless a gift. The donor has made a decision to transfer assets to your organization for a general or specific purpose, and this is more often than not a very significant planned gift. A donor that is properly recognized and thanked may well consider making additional gifts in the future, or perhaps even increasing the size of the commitment at a later date. Even "anonymous" gifts should be properly recognized. It is usually appropriate for the chief executive officer and perhaps one or more board members to send letters of thanks to an anonymous donor. It is always a nice touch for the planned giving officer to send a handwritten note of thanks on proper stationery. Also, the personalization of the acknowledgment process can be extremely important to the donor. Recognition is normally based on the full fair-market value of the gift. There is really no such thing as a "discount value" in recognizing generosity.

DRAFTING AN OPERATING PLAN

Assume that your organization has become much more sophisticated about planned giving, and its officers and staff have established procedures and taken initiatives that will lead to a whole new kind of increased philanthropy. Now is the time to draft a planned giving operating plan that will include all of the essential details and dates of the key steps in your program for the following year. Drafting such a plan is much more than an exercise in accountability. In committing your ideas and your program to paper, you are encouraged to think big. How many donor trips will you be able to make during the course of the year? When you are traveling, should you plan on seeing three prospects a day, or can you manage a larger number? How many prospects a year would that be? Have you coordinated your travel plans with mailings and the time necessary for follow-up from the mailings? Are other major gifts officers aware of your program, and can they participate and make their own contributions to its success? Are you making the best use of your available resources and staff? Is your marketing plan truly imaginative, and effective in capturing the attention of your constituency? Are you sharing ideas and plans with other successful organizations so that you can strengthen your plan? Perhaps most important of all, do you have a strategic approach to planned giving, and will your approach help you to focus on those individuals most likely to make significant gifts to your organization? These are all questions of experience and judgment, and as the program develops, the art of planned giving comes to the forefront.

In evaluating your results, neither a "soft and fuzzy" approach nor a "by the numbers" approach will give you the information you really need. To sustain success in a planned giving program for a period of longer than 5 years, it is obviously essential that your plans have depth and purposefulness. In all of your efforts, it should be apparent that planned giving helps to support the mission of your organization, now and in the future. Planned giving should be understood as being neither "technical" nor "deferred." The goal of planned giving, and of your planned giving program, is to make it as easy as possible for individuals to make the largest gift that they possibly can based on their involvement with your organization and the assets that they have available for philanthropic giving.

ADVANCED ISSUES IN PLANNED GIVING

The Planned Giving Advisory Committee

It is conventional wisdom that one of the first things that you need to do when establishing a planned giving program is to recruit a planned giving advisory committee. The usual thinking is that such a committee should include an attorney, a CPA, a real estate agent, a life insurance sales person, and other professionals who can advise the planned giving officer on gift situations as they arise. In my experience, most of these committees are comprised of between 10 and 12 individuals, although there are some that number actually over 100 in membership. I know of one such committee that included the full range of professional estate planners and financial advisors, but that did not include a single person who had put the philanthropy in his or her own estate plans. The members of this group were not donors to the organization, and would never consider making a large gift for any purpose to the organization. The chairman of the committee was highly regarded, and was a leader in his profession, but he believed that his serving on the committee was his gift to the organization. Such committees require a great deal of staff time to provide them with adequate support, plan meetings, produce literature and agendas, and related activities. The organization, the members of the committee, and especially the planned giving officer were extremely frustrated by having to deal with the existence of this committee. It was actually a hindrance to furthering the planned giving effort.

One of the nation's leading capital campaign consultants, who has managed several billion dollar campaigns, suggests that you only need five individuals as volunteers to conduct a billion dollar campaign. The emphasis for him is on leadership and capability, not to mention dedication to the organization and willingness to work hard and long. If you decide that you need and must have a planned giving committee, you should consider recruiting only those individuals with strong ties to your organization who are or surely will become generous donors and loyal contributors. The committee should be seen as existing to help identify and cultivate prospects, and to lend technical advice only on those occasions when it is really needed. If you have the perfect person to chair such a small group, you may be successful. My advice is to give up any idea of having such a committee unless you are confident that it will meet all of the criteria needed to make it a sure success.

Working with a Consultant

There are many fine consultants in planned giving, and many of the most successful programs engage these consultants to work with them in establishing the program and in helping to keep it fresh and vital. Some consultants specialize in the instruments of planned giving from a legal or estate planning point of view, and others are especially good at marketing and promoting the concept of planned giving to a wider audience. It is perfectly legitimate for an organization considering the establishment of a planned giving program to bring in an experienced and reliable consultant to do a planned giving audit and feasibility study. This will give the CEO and members of the board enough information to decide whether they should go ahead with such a program. In ordinary circumstances, the planned giving consultant should not solicit prospects for your organization and should not become a sort of "visiting" staff member. Once a planned giving program is up and running, it may be useful to have a consultant come in two or three times a year to meet with staff members and brainstorm new initiatives and other ideas.

Another alternative is to have the planned giving officer, perhaps in the company of the vice president for development or CEO of the organization, attend an advanced giving seminar that provides the opportunity for idea exchange and questioning. It is always a refreshing and motivating experience to see what creative ideas have been developed by others, and to learn new perspectives and approaches. You should know whether or not that radio campaign for gift annuities being run by a major institution in your town is really working. And are there any new ideas on how to conduct estate planning seminars for your constituency? You may have other agenda issues that could be satisfied by attending such seminars. I know of one CEO who attended a few planned giving seminars in order to identify candidates for an open planned giving director position in his organization. His executive search was successful.

Mission and Charitable Intent

Planned giving is sometimes wrongly promoted as a form of investment vehicle, such as a mutual fund. Some organizations have developed advertising strategies that emphasize only the tax benefits of planned giving, and essentially offer potential donors new methods of dodging taxes and increasing their income. Such an approach completely ignores the fundamentals of charitable giving. Very few donors give money in order to receive deductions and evade taxes. If there are such donors, they are going to shop their gift among several philanthropies to see where they can get the best bargain in terms of income payout and perhaps other special treatment. These donors may have no special interest in your organization or its future, and are not deeply motivated to give something back to society. Any approach that seems "too good to be true" is probably something that you should avoid at all costs. The National Committee on Planned Giving and the National Society of Fund Raising Executives have codes of ethics that will help to guide professional staff members, trustees, and other volunteers. The codes of ethics of these organizations are taken very seriously, and should be endorsed by you and your organization.

Planned giving programs serve the greater purposes of philanthropy and fundraising in very effective ways. It is a very basic human need to pass assets from an individual who has some accumulated wealth to either a philanthropy or to natural heirs. Very often this process does not work in the best interests of the individual or of society. In the December 27, 1999, issue of *Forbes*, an article entitled "Willful Omission" begins by stating the problem:

> It's bad enough when a loved one dies, and it will get even worse if the person died without a will. Dying intestate leaves heirs with a bundle of legal, administrative and tax headaches. And even if you get an inheritance, there might be little you can do about crushing tax consequences. These nightmares notwithstanding, more than half of American adults die without a will. They have ranged from presidents, including Abraham Lincoln

and Ulysses S. Grant, to businessmen, like Howard Hughes who died leaving $2 billion, no valid will and a 15-year legal tussle. (Sanders, 1999, p. 252)

The article continues,

Why do so many otherwise thoughtful people fail to plan their estate? Procrastination. Thoughtlessness. Or maybe just fear of mortality.

Planned giving addresses the need of individuals to dispose of their assets in the most appropriate and thoughtful way. The opportunities made available through planned giving allow people to become philanthropists while helping to assure that their estate plans will take maximum advantage of the tax laws and meet their personal objectives.

INSTRUMENTS AND METHODS OF PLANNED GIVING

The Bequest

Bequests to philanthropic organizations are fundamental to the health and future of the not-for-profit sector. Some of America's leading arts, educational, and healthcare organizations were founded through the bequest of a thoughtful individual. The endowments that support organizations such as hospitals, universities, youth organizations, and art museums are formed principally through philanthropic bequests.

Wills are simple but powerful documents. It takes only a few lines to leave millions of dollars to a philanthropy if the person is sufficiently wealthy and motivated to give. A bequest may specify an amount of money, such as $25,000, or a specific kind of property, such as real estate, shares in a company, or an art collection. Since many people are not really sure what their net worth will be when they die, they may prefer to leave the philanthropy a percentage of the residuary estate. The residuary estate is what is left in the estate after all bills have been paid, bequests of specific amounts have been paid, and other costs taken out. I know of one woman whose estate grew from about $5 million to $50 million during the decades while she had become mentally incompetent. Fortunately, her estate provided that one-half of the total residuary estate would go to each of two philanthropies. What would have happened if she had left each philanthropy $2.5 million? Another possibility is for an individual to leave the entire residuary estate to a single philanthropy. This is usually an extraordinary act of generosity.

Life-Income Agreements

Life-income agreements include the well-known charitable remainder trusts, pooled income funds, and gift annuities. Life-income agreements pay the donor, and often the donor's spouse, an income for life that is either a specific annual amount or a variable annual amount. There are many tax advantages in making gifts through these agreements, including an immediate income tax deduction for a portion of the gift based on the donor's age, the payout of the life income agreement, and the number of beneficiaries. Generally, the older the donor the greater the amount of annual payment and the higher the deduction. Life-income agreements are irrevocable. That is, the gift cannot be taken back. Because the gift is completed when the agreement is funded, the donor is entitled to the above tax deductions. In most cases, the philanthropy will not benefit from the principal of the trust until the death of the last income beneficiary. For the philanthropy, the benefit is deferred.

Life-income agreements are very attractive to donors and to philanthropies. The donor enjoys tax benefits, and may receive increased income because of the nature of the charitable agreement. The philanthropy enjoys the benefit of receiving an irrevocable gift that will eventually add significant resources to support the future of the organization. In addition, recognition can be given to the donor or donors at the time the gift is made, so that the individuals can be thanked for their philanthropy during their lifetimes.

One of the principal benefits of charitable remainder trusts is the significant reduction or elimination of federal gift and estates taxes. As increasing wealth is held in the hands of individuals, the more important it becomes to shelter family assets from taxation. The federal estate tax, for example, can take 55% (as of January 1, 1993) of all assets in excess of a certain amount.

When a single individual, or husband and wife, are the beneficiaries of a charitable life income trust, gift and estate taxes are completely avoided for the assets placed in the charitable trust. When children or other individuals receive all or part of the income from such charitable trusts, there is a significant reduction in the gift or estate taxes that would otherwise be payable; of course, if capital gains are distributed as part of the annual income, they would be taxed along with ordinary income. A charitable gift planning officer can provide accurate calculations that will graphically illustrate the extent of the tax benefits made available through charitable remainder trusts.

A comprehensive estate plan for a donor or a family will take into consideration all of the tax and other benefits of philanthropic giving through charitable trusts, bequests, and other methods. The nature of the assets held, and the intentions of the donor(s) are key to a successfully executed estate plan.

When a donor has selected a philanthropy to support through planned giving, the donor often meets with the planned giving officers representing the organization, and may encourage his legal and tax advisers to meet with these planned giving officers as well. A team approach should be a very efficient and effective way to maximize the tax benefits of charitable giving.

Fixed Income Agreements

There are four basic kinds of life-income agreements that fall into two categories:

Gift Annuities

Gift annuities are the most simple kind of life-income agreement, and have been popular for many generations. A gift annuity agreement can usually be drafted on one side of one sheet of paper, and requires very little information from the donor. Unique among life-income agreements, the charitable gift annuity is not a form of trust, but rather a contract between the philanthropy and the donor in which the philanthropy agrees to pay the donor a fixed amount for the life of the donor based on the receipt of a gift. By law, there can be no more than two income beneficiaries.

Payout rates on gift annuities can be based upon the suggested rates published by the American Council on Gift Annuities, a national organization of philanthropies that offer gift annuities to their supporters. A new gift annuity can be funded with as little as $10,000, and sometimes $5,000, making this a very attractive vehicle for people with limited resources. Because the income is fixed, the gift annuity is especially attractive to older contributors who receive higher income, some of which is free of taxation for the life expectancy of the donor (as established by federal tables). Since there are some capital gains implications with gift annuities, they may not be the best vehicle when the donor is funding the agreement with highly appreciated assets. An experienced planned giving officer can "run the calculations" to see if a gift annuity is a good option.

Since you cannot add to a gift annuity, donors very often create new gift annuities from time to time. In my experience, the largest number of gift annuities created by a single donor was 18. Perhaps this donor is still creating new gift annuities.

Since the philanthropy is liable for making the gift annuity payments, some philanthropies would not feel comfortable accepting gift annuities larger than $500,000, and perhaps not as large as this. If a donor were to live to be, for example, 110 years old, the philanthropy might possibly lose money on a gift annuity with this individual. This would be a very rare case, and none has ever come to my attention. Your organization's financial officers may be very concerned, however.

The Charitable Remainder Annuity Trust

The charitable remainder annuity trust is a much more complicated vehicle, and requires the careful scrutiny of experienced attorneys and planned giving officers. The trust is usually funded with a larger gift, usually $50,000 to $100,000 as a minimum. The donor and the philanthropy agree upon a payout rate which is a percentage of the trust assets at the time the gift is made. For a variety of reasons, it is important that this percentage not be set too high. A charitable remainder annuity trust can "run dry" if the payout rates exceed the income generated by the trust. Since most organizations are now fairly sophisticated about managing this kind of trust, such a disastrous consequence would not ordinarily occur.

A donor to a charitable remainder annuity trust enjoys the avoidance of capital gains taxes when the gift is made, and an immediate income tax deduction based on the age and payout rate of the donor or donors, and a specific amount of income for life. Since the trust instrument is a complex document, the trust can be tailored more carefully to the personal needs and circumstances of the donor. The charitable remainder annuity trust remains one of the most popular life-income agreements available.

Variable Income Agreements

Pooled Income Funds

Pooled income funds are very popular during times of high inflation, high interest rates, and high payout rates by money market funds. Pooled income funds must distribute all of the income that they earn on an annual basis to the donors who have made gifts to the fund. Gifts from all donors to the fund are "pooled" together as one investment portfolio, and most pooled income funds are invested for the highest possible income.

Some philanthropies have more than one pooled income fund, and invest one for high income and another for low income and possible growth in principal. The pooled income fund offers all of the income and capital gains tax advantages of charitable remainder trusts. An individual can usually make a gift to a pooled income fund of $10,000, or sometimes $5,000, as an initial contribution. Donors may make additional contributions to the same fund over a period of years, and this is a very simple procedure. Pooled income funds were in their glory during the high inflation years of the 1970s.

Charitable Remainder Unitrust

The charitable remainder unitrust is the most flexible of all of the life-income agreements. Here again, the donor or donors receive income for life, tax advantages, and the avoidance of capital gains taxes on gifts of appreciated property. The payout rate is a percentage of the total assets in the trust *as calculated yearly*. If a donor is receiving 7% of the trust assets in income, the initial-year payout will be 7% of the assets that are contributed to the trust. If the trust grows in the second year, the income payout will be higher. On the other hand, if the investments in the trust result in a smaller principal, the income payout will be lower that year. Younger donors in their 50s or early 60s may prefer the charitable remainder unitrust because of the possible increase in principal during the expected lifetimes of the donor or donors. In addition, a special variation on the unitrust may be used to receive assets such as real estate or buildings that will need to be sold to produce income producing liquid assets for investment in the trust.

Life-income agreements are the primary focus of many planned giving programs. Since they offer both immediate and future tax benefits to the contributors, they are extremely attractive as options for philanthropic giving. They encourage donors to consider much larger gifts, and can be used as the entire commitment of a donor to an organization, or as part of a complex gift that might be part cash, part charitable remainder trust, and part bequest, for example.

Charitable Lead Trust

The charitable lead trust received its name because the philanthropy "leads" in receiving income. The purpose of establishing a charitable lead trust, either a unitrust or an annuity trust in form of payment, is to transfer assets from the donor or donors to another generation, usually children, and sometimes grandchildren. Since the philanthropy begins receiving yearly contributions from a lead trust, it is not a deferred gift, but a planned gift in its true sense. Lead trusts are especially attractive to people who have total assets of at least $2–3 million, and perhaps at least $5 million. By avoiding or minimizing capital gains taxes and gift taxes in passing property, the donor can assure that children or other individuals will receive the principal of the trust at a later date, usually at least 10 or 15 years after the creation of the trust. The longer the period of the trust, and the higher the payout rate to philanthropy, the greater the tax advantages. Charitable lead trusts are most attractive when interest rates are very low because the deduction tables are related to monthly interest rates as calculated by the government. Most philanthropies, even the largest and most sophisticated, receive very few gifts through charitable lead trusts.

Life Insurance

The best kind of life insurance gift is the one that transfers a fully paid-up policy with a redemption value to a philanthropy. This is really a form of outright property gift, but is usually handled by the planned giving office. However, most gifts of life insurance to philanthropies are made by donors who take out a life insurance policy and name the philanthropy as a beneficiary. Because insurance policy gifts may be regulated by state law, it is always important to be aware of individual state laws and restrictions.

Some organizations have encouraged every member of their board of trustees to take out such a policy. This can be complicated when the individuals who establish such life insurance policies feel that they have "made their gift" to the philanthropy, and decide not to make other kinds of gifts to capital campaigns or annual campaigns. This can be very costly to a philanthropy, and can undermine the basis of its support and hinder its ability to conduct campaigns. A gift of a life insurance policy to a philanthropy can be of great value, but a plan to market life insurance gifts to a broad constituency within a philanthropy should be thought through very carefully.

Real Estate

Gifts of real estate can be of extraordinary value to a philanthropy. Some large universities even employ attorneys specializing in dealing with this kind of gift. However, receiving the gift of real estate is more complicated than it was several years ago. For one thing, it is now necessary to conduct an environmental analysis of the property. If a philanthropy were to accept a piece of property, and later find out that there were hidden toxic wastes on the property, it could be sued for owning such a toxic waste dump, or could be liable to have all of the toxic waste removed. This could cost millions of dollars, and make the gift seem completely insignificant. Unfortunately, this is not a theoretical question. I have actually seen cases where an environmental analysis resulted in the donor deciding not to make a gift of real estate to the philanthropy. This can be embarrassing both to the donor and to the philanthropy. Nonetheless, gifts of real estate should ordinarily be encouraged, and planned giving officers should be aware of the appropriate steps to take in receiving such gifts. One experienced planned giving officer keeps a complete checklist of all the steps to go through when handling such a gift.

SUMMARY

Planned giving should be an integral component of any major development effort, and is intricately interwoven with major gift fundraising. Just as with other components, it is important to have the expertise in the details of planned given among development staff or consultants. Systematic goal-setting and program planning for any planned giving component of the development activities will enhance the results.

REFERENCES

Dunlop, D. R. (1986). Special concerns of major gift fund-raising. In W. Rowland (Ed.), *Handbook of institutional advancement* (pp. 322–336). San Francisco: Jossey-Bass.

Odendahl, T. (Ed.). (1987). *America's wealthy and the future of foundations.* New York: The Foundation Center.

Sanders, A. (1999). Willful omission. *Forbes, 164*(15), 252–254.

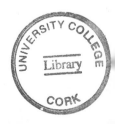

8

Foundation and Corporate Development

MYRNA J. PETERSEN

T he area of fundraising that has experienced the most profound metamorphosis in the last two decades is that of foundation and corporate funds development. The transformation was spurred in the early 1980s when the philanthropic community, its assets buoyed by a soaring stock market, stepped forward to address the nation's social and health needs in the wake of the retreat of government funding. It was inevitable that the increased competition for philanthropic dollars would result in the growing sophistication of grant makers, and of corporate and foundation development as a profession. In 1998 alone (1999 figures were not yet available as this chapter went to press), U.S. foundations gave away no less than $17.09 billion—a 22.9% increase over the previous year, and the third year of double digit growth in giving* (AAFRC Press Release, 1999). Schools that have underutilized this resource in the past would be wise to consider foundations as fresh constituents and potential partners in achieving shared goals. Individuals will always be a school's primary resource for gifts (77.3% of giving + 7.8% in bequests), but foundation grants (typically 9.8% of all philanthropic giving from independent and community foundations—and close to one-fifth of private contributions, if giving for religion is excluded*), together with corporate giving (now down to 5.1% after a peak at 6.5% in the mid-1980s*),

---

* All data reported here are from the AAFRC May 1999 Press Release.

76

can also push a school toward its fundraising goals. Significantly, the cultivation of working relationships with major foundations and corporations can advance a school's ability to improve health care interventions, better prepare health professionals, contribute to the development of policy, and position the school to recruit quality faculty and students.

To understand what grantsmanship is today is to know what is no longer. As recently as the 20th century (!), grant-seeking was primarily the endeavor of academic researchers—faculty accustomed to the federal grant process. Seasoned academicians well remember the heyday of the 1960s when funds could be obtained by mailing one generic proposal to many prospective funders and then simply waiting for the checks to come in. That "shotgun" approach lost its effectiveness (and gained a reputation as "double-dipping") as grantmakers themselves became better regulated, more sophisticated—and less isolated. Today, to keep abreast of the hundreds of requests that come in the door, both foundations and corporations have program officers, who are often program experts themselves, to screen and evaluate the worthiness of requests and make recommendations to trustees. In their desire to be more knowledgeable and proactive in creating initiatives and effecting policy, trustees and program officers now enjoy a network of formal and informal communications through local funders' forums, regional associations, and national affinity groups. In short, foundation people talk with each other, and they are a font of information. They know about current grants and new proposals, and they have the ear of civic and academic leaders engaged in planning future programs. In any given city, it is likely that a program officer will know more about what is happening in your program area than you do. What a resource!

Because it is a funder's market today, funders can and do demand requests that are visionary and that are tailored specifically to their mission and to the goals they hope to achieve through the distribution of their assets. What is more, they want to know that they are investing in an institution that has the track record and capacity to carry off the program well. For a sizeable project, the funder wants assurance that the individual responsible for the program (the principal investigator) is totally committed to meeting the stated objectives, that the proposal is being submitted with the knowledge (i.e., clearance) and conceptual support of the requesting institution, and that the impact of the grant will be diffused via collaborations and the dissemination of knowledge learned through the funded project. Funders do not work in a vacuum, and neither should you. What is exciting is the degree to which grantmakers and grantseekers have come to work in partnership with one another, and this is as true with corporate development as it is in foundation development. So how does one tailor a request to meet the funder's expectations?

Grant-seeking from an entity is similar to soliciting individual contributions in that the success of the "ask" is directly related to how "sold" the prospect is on your product. The better the product, the more lucrative the payoff. Yes, there is a high degree of salesmanship in development, and the most successful salespersons are those who know the features and benefits of their own product—and who are cognizant of what their customers desire and how they think. The good news is that this information is available and easier to access now than ever before. Virtually every funding source has funding guidelines and a tax filing, and that information is available to the public. A foundation's IRS return, Form 990-PF, can be requested through The Foundation Center libraries. This provides a listing of each private foundation's basic financial data, officers' names, and a complete grants list.

When available, the more revealing source is a funder's Annual Report, as this narrative usually notes the original source of the funds, the mission, the current funding initiatives, examples of recent grants, contributions guidelines and contact persons, and the names of trustees, officers, distribution committees, and professional staff. Knowing the source of the money and the history of the founder or the foundation offers insight to why the mission is what it is, and can help you to anticipate what proposals may be of interest. Like the constitution, a foundation's mission is difficult to change even with legal action, so even if their funding programs change from year to year, you will always know the purpose of the existence of each and every foundation.

Important reading is found in the introductory pages of an annual report. In addition to promotional highlights, the message from the chairman or president of a foundation, or from the chief executive of a corporation, reveals personal or institutional commitments, goals the entity hopes to achieve through its funding investments, and shifts in focus. If your proposed program is compatible with the funder's mission, if you feel a kinship with the goals and aspirations of the foundation's leadership, and if your project appears to fall within the funding guidelines, you may well be onto a viable prospect. If not, do not waste your time (or theirs) in pursuit of something they could not fund even if you were their best friend. It is noteworthy that the flexibility enjoyed by an individual or a corporation in giving away money is not possible for a foundation that, by law, must give grants that fall within the limitations of their own mission and guidelines. Do not be dismayed, as research on any given day will bring to the surface alternative funding sources that may be an even better fit for what you want to do.

Doing your homework is key to matching your project to a funding entity, but you will not live long enough to read the annual report of every corporation and foundation. Fortunately, there are excellent (and free) sources at your disposal, both in the library and on the Internet, and at the top of the list is "The Foundation Centers." On the World Wide Web, simply keying in http://fdncenter.org opens the door to a world of information—everything you want to know and more about how to get a project funded, including links to Web sites of grant makers. The Foundation Center has five libraries—in Atlanta, Cleveland, New York, San Francisco, and Washington, DC—where staff are available to train grantseekers in how to use the many published and electronic resources available, both at these five libraries and also at the 200 Cooperating Collections that are affiliated with The Foundation Center. Another Web site, http//www.philanthropy.com, offers access to portions of *The Chronicle of Philanthropy.* Previously available solely as a pricy bi-weekly tabloid-format newspaper, this comprehensive resource keeps abreast of recently awarded grants as well as fundraising trends and issues. Much of the *Chronicle's* online information is available only to subscribers. Nevertheless, the free portion includes articles and a list of upcoming grant deadlines and conferences—as well as headlines of articles that you can look up in hard copy at the library. Not to be discounted are the daily papers, where current news coverage is at times complemented by articles on philanthropy and donor profiles. Use that "daily" as a launch pad for ideas—what can you do to help resolve the problems of today?

While this chapter concentrates on resources freely available to the general public, be aware that a variety of funding source databases exist in subscription format, and the advantage of those is the ability to do keyword searches (your school or library may subscribe to some of these, so inquire at your research office or ask the development staff about what resources may be available to faculty). In addition, newsletters such as *Foundation Giving Watch*, the *Corporate Giving Watch*, and the *Health Care Grants and Contracts Weekly* publish helpful and informational funding alerts that can effectively shortcut the search process and send you directly to new Calls for Proposals. Appendix B includes a listing of directories to lead you through the search process. In general, available to assist you through the maze of sources is an array of how-to books, workshops, and Web sites written/hosted by trustees, program officers, and academicians, all of whom are quite happy to share what has worked for them and what to avoid. Grant-seeking is more of an art than a science, so take heed, as there are pitfalls to be avoided. But common sense and solid effort will take you far, and for as much as there is to learn about this process, there are plenty of experienced people ready, willing, and able to help with questions that arise. Following are some hints to get you started.

The most commonly used reference for specific foundations, and one that is especially useful to new grantseekers, is *The Foundation Directory*, compiled annually by The Foundation Center. In hard copy, this is a three-inch thick listing of 8,000+ foundations providing annual grants of $200,000 or more (a companion publication, *The Foundation Directory Part 2*, lists sources that make grants in the range of $50,000 to $200,000). The *Directory* is arranged alphabetically by the states in which the foundations reside, and contains all the basic information you need to know to determine whether or not this is an entity to be pursued further: name, address, telephone, contact person, and printed materials available from the foundation (look for newsletters from sources that match your interests), date established, donors, officers and trustees, areas of giving, types of grants, assets and high-low grant amounts, limitations, application information, and representative grants. Other resources such as the *Foundation Reporter* (Taft) include foundation philosophy and a contributions analysis—in-depth information that is valuable once you have narrowed the search. Unless you are seeking in-depth information on a particular foundation, the first place to turn in this or any directory is the Index, to conduct what on the World Wide Web would be a keyword search. Go to the Subject Index to see which foundations fund the topic of your project, and be prepared to get creative if none of the subject names coincide exactly with your topic. Or, turn to the Types of Support Index to see which entities fund equipment, for example, or perhaps endowments or capital campaigns. What is helpful is that the listings within these indexes are also grouped by state (there is also a section for international giving). While entities in bold face make grants on a national, regional, or international basis, explore your own state first, as your organization is a natural constituent of funding sources that reside within (or have a major presence in) a radius of your locale.

People give to people, and this axiom is true even for foundations and corporations, whose checks must be written to the school and not to individual faculty. It is advantageous and fortunate for a school when a dean or faculty member has a high-level linkage to a corporation or foundation that has evolved out of that individual's academic or professional endeavors. Whether a researcher or community clinician, there is nothing that speaks more strongly than demonstrated knowledge and successful practice. But even for the novice, with resourcefulness and persistence, contact with, say, a sales representative can eventually lead to funding if the faculty member has a program that is of interest to that source. Development officers can be useful in drawing out and helping to facilitate those linkages, and they also can be a godsend to busy faculty by doing the work of researching and identifying prospects. Further, because repeat or multi-year grants are difficult to get, the development officer can serve as a facilitator in guiding the philanthropic cultivation and stewardship necessary to maintain an ongoing relationship with a funding source.

It is of paramount importance to know who the contact person is at the foundation and who the program officers are. Cultivate these relationships, because if a program interests them, these individuals will reveal a surprising amount of information that will be of assistance in the proposal process—and they may also point the way to alternative funding sources. In searching the directories (most directories include an alphabetical listing of donors, officers and trustees of the foundations) and Web sites of funders, also watch for the names of trustees and officers, and look for who is on the distribution committee. Some of these may be persons who are highly visible and known as the "movers and shakers" in the community. If the faculty member writing the proposal or the leadership of the school shares common interests and goals with the leadership of the funding institution, that may be the basis for a mutually rewarding relationship. In some closely held corporations, a well-established comfort level could possibly allow you to bypass the complex maneuvering that may otherwise lie between you and the check. For that reason, "who knows who" is an appropriate question for the dean and for the school's board of trustees. The development officer can also help to ferret out connections that faculty or alumni may have with foundations and corporations through business or professional affiliations—or through family ties. Used with discretion, personal connections can be helpful in developing partnerships between the school and a community's funding sources. Also, exploring these connections helps draw the individual providing the linkage closer to the school and its mission (individual gifts fundraisers take note, as a school can greatly expand its relationship with these individuals by adding a mix of informational correspondence to the thank-you notes). Regardless, in grant-seeking, a school's strong suit will always be the credibility of its faculty and leadership and the strength and urgency of the proposed concept.

Your goal is to have a conversation with someone knowledgeable at the funding source that you are targeting—preferably the program officer in a sizeable foundation or, in a smaller fund, the executive director or grants administrator, if not the donor family. In a privately held corporate entity, this may be the chief executive officer, or in larger organizations, the vice president for community affairs. (For convenience, this chapter uses the term "program officer" to cover all bases). If a foundation's Call for Proposals posts an informational session prior to the proposal deadline date, by all means attend this meeting, as it is an excellent opportunity to meet the program officers, to get some of your questions answered—and to see what your competition is for that initiative. Prepare for your conversation with the funder in two ways: first, read published materials and scan the Web to learn how your project fits into the funder's mission. Next, even when it is not required, prepare a Concept Paper. The power of the written word—committing your idea to paper—is the first step toward realizing your project. Writing forces you to bring your own thoughts into focus, and within the academic setting, this text will also help others to more fully grasp and appreciate your ideas and strategies. For those working as a team, the negotiation of what goes into the draft is a necessary process that will coalesce both the team and the project. Once formalized, the concept paper serves as the starting point for discussion with potential partners, and it also becomes the basis for negotiation for institutional clearance to submit a proposal to a particular funder (necessary because many foundations will entertain only one proposal from an institution in a grant cycle). Keep the development staff fully informed of your intentions so they can assist in the clearance process. Sharing your concept paper with the program officer provides a basis for discussion, and saves time for both you and the officer if the content is not of interest. In fact, a concept paper is required by many foundations today as a screening device, followed by an invitation for a proposal if they feel the concept is worthy of development.

Regardless of how formal or informal the process is, whenever possible, request feedback from the program officer before you launch into a full-blown proposal: What in particular attracted them to your program? Is there any aspect that is weak and should either be eliminated altogether or strengthened in some way? Do they have any questions for you? Listen carefully to the program officer for key words and issues that will help focus your writing. Savor this conversation, as it may be the beginning of a long relationship.

This may be the best place to scratch the surface about the complexities of courting a corporation, even though that could be a chapter unto itself. The strategy has a key similarity to that used in cultivating individual gifts: you must win the trust and the heart before you can benefit from the largesse of this prospect. Corporate development differs from a foundation in that the opportunities are often fleeting and the process may be elusive and not as lucrative as you would have hoped. Survival and success in today's complex business world demands a nimble operation, so once your foot is in the door, be prepared to provide quick turnaround on requests for information. Then listen carefully in order to seize the moment appropriately when interest surfaces. At the same time, the business community has long been at the forefront of strategic planning and the building of partnerships for mutual gain. The result is a prevalence of rich environments largely untapped for long-term positioning, and time devoted to this level of cultivation can result in a fulfilling long-term relationship. The trick is to figure out the linkages between your business and theirs, and to do that requires awareness of market needs and "out of the box" thinking. Again, homework helps. The corporation itself may appear to be tremendously wealthy, but that wealth may already be earmarked for an upcoming acquisition (or for fighting off one), or in the case of conversions, the establishment of a foundation with philanthropic motives may be in the offing. Above all, you are dealing with people who enjoy camaraderie, whose livelihood is based on a combination of risk and trust, and who revel in the intrigue of the business game. This is where well-selected board members can be of tremendous assistance to your school's efforts. These individuals can feed you information that is not within your normal scope of knowledge, and help you to prepare the prospect and determine when to make an "ask"—and tell you which pocket to aim for.

So which corporation do you target, and which of its pockets do you aim for? Think local, again, as you are the natural constituent of those whose backyard you sit in. Today's exhibitor or vendor may be tomorrow's sponsor of your event or scholarship, so faculty should take careful note of what products they use and their product representatives or regional sales managers. Similar to the case of the foundation, your ticket of admission is to identify and respond to a need, but in the corporate world, it is less altruistic and unabashedly known as "What's in it for me?" (that is, for the corporation, not for you—although there obviously must be something in it for you, too, or you should not be there). The sales division, a business's first line of offense, operates in closest proximity to the "bottom line," and this is where need can be most quickly identified and satisfied. For this reason, decisions can be made on the spot if your ask is within that "rep's" or division's discretionary budget. Your phone call (or a time-consuming series of calls, if your school still needs to build vendor relationships) could result in a positive response if you are realistic in your request. Ask for what is needed, discuss what is possible, and consider accepting a product as an option or supplement to a monetary gift. In-kind gifts are attributable to a school's fundraising attainment as long as the gift is accompanied by a letter from the donor stating the value of the gift. In the interest of stimulating sales, it is not unusual for a publishing sales rep to give a faculty member a complimentary copy of a new textbook, or for a school to be given an educational video or CD (request a multisite institutional license to go with it). The more substantial the request, the more likely the need for a meeting and a follow-up request in writing. A close relationship coupled with a ripe sales market could result in new state-of-the-art equipment for an entire classroom or laboratory. In other words, the budget for contributions does exist—especially if a corporation can be convinced that association with your school offers attractive exposure. Again, do your homework. For example, how many health professionals will use the lab or workshop for which you want corporate support? Or, how important is the conference content and participant profile to the corporation? Once interest is captured, be clear about what you are agreeing to, and be mindful that expectations set with a sponsor this year may establish a precedent that is difficult to change in subsequent years (e.g., don't give away so many tickets to your event that it negates the value of the gift). If the value of what the donor receives in exchange is equal to or in excess of the value of the gift to you, it is not a charitable gift. Ask your legal counsel if you have any questions regarding the charitable nature of a gift, as there is a fine distinction between advertising (e.g., use of logo) and support of a program (e.g., an acknowledged gift). Regardless of the value of the gift, it could be a one-time dole if you fail to respond with the same stewardship that you would if you had received a large grant. At the very least, send an acknowledgment letter and, when warranted, a report on how the gift was used and how it was valued by students and faculty. Such documentation will provide a record of the transaction for future reference.

A friendly relationship with a corporation's sales division can lead to larger opportunities through its marketing division—the people responsible for promoting the name and logo of that entity. This is the division that responds to arguments for visibility or positioning, and it is where exciting partnerships can be crafted for the exploration of markets where neither of you has gone before. Will that corporation benefit by associating its name with your institution? How much publicity can you/should you promise to give to their gift (to put that into perspective, consider your own advertising costs), and for how long? Will linkage with that corporate name/logo benefit your school, or can you at least live with it comfortably? If the gift is significant, these are questions that require discussion with your school's dean, the institution's president, and the office of communications. By and large, though, the benefits will be mutual, and again your trusted board members can help steer you to the most likely prospects.

If you do engage in a joint endeavor (not only with corporations, but also for foundation grant collaborations), it is not only desirable, but also necessary, when partnerships are involved, to confirm in writing what has been agreed to verbally. This document, written on the institution's letterhead and signed by the executive, may be a simple statement of agreement, or a more complex document, outlining each partner's responsibilities.

What can you do while trying to attract more corporate participation to your board? Start by reading the business pages and attending major functions of your city's business leaders. Ask questions to learn about the corporate culture and what is important to the individuals who reside in that sector. Today, many corporations encourage their employees to volunteer, including everything from painting a community building to sitting on the boards of not-for-profits. In the same vein, they also can arrange to provide equipment, technical assistance, or administrative advice (these are in-kind gifts, so ask the corporation to set a value and convey this to you in a letter). Chosen wisely, the added value of having a volunteer on your board is that the corporate perspective can stimulate the real-world relevancy of your educational program, and this is critical to any academic endeavor. Aim high (for example, well-connected CEOs and VPs for Patient Services) so that decision makers are at your table to foster collaborations and attract other high hitters. Engaging leadership in meaningful consultation and discussion, coupled with cultivation strategies, can lead the way to the other pocket of a corporation: individual major gifts, ranging from scholarships to endowed chairs or named centers of excellence. But do not assume you will receive a major gift just because the capacity exists. The heart must be there, as well. Like a marriage, solid commitment rarely comes without consistent courting and a lot of give along with the take.

Overall, confidence in your own school's worth and capabilities must be coupled with patience when pursuing a corporate relationship. Be direct in identifying mutual and respective benefits of the proposed long-term partnership, and bold and visionary in articulating the nature of a new product, market, or relationship, and do not be afraid to discuss issues of concern. What appears to be off-again-on-again interest may simply reflect market fluctuations, or if the company is in a huge growth spurt, it is possible that no one at the corporation has time to piece the partnership together for you, and that they may be hoping you will take that lead. That brings us back to the power of drafting a concept paper or a preliminary memorandum of agreement. By giving your prospect something to respond to, you allow them to assume the position of offering you guidance—that is, helping you to shape your "ask," which is exactly where you want to be!

Advice from a program officer, trustee, or corporate official may not always be what you want to hear because it may mean more work than you had intended. If you do not understand a comment or have questions, now is the time to ask, as that advice is coming from someone who has information that you could not know; such as what other proposals are coming across their desk, or what initiatives they have coming down the road that you should try to position yourself for. You could be asked to reduce the budget (if so, adjust your objectives accordingly) or to find matching funds. A junior faculty member may be advised to partner with a more senior faculty member. A research method may be questioned, or a project may be found to be more ambitious than what can be done in the time and budget proposed. A clinical practice team may be advised to add an interdisciplinary component. It may be recommended that a Caucasian faculty member include a minority faculty member on the research team when that minority group is the target for data collection. A school might be told to form an advisory board to gain the support of the community and ensure that it is acting in their best interests. What you do to "regroup" and act on advice—or to simply seek funding elsewhere—depends on your school's program priorities and other existing relationships. Still, advice from program officers is a genuine effort to help you do what you need to do to get funded, so take it into consideration, and incorporate it into your project if feasible.

One factor that should always be kept in mind, and one that the program officer can help you identify, is the decision makers—the individual(s) who will read and put a dollar value on your proposal. Is it a nurse, who will understand your program intuitively? Not likely. Is it a physician who is skeptical of nurses? Possibly, but then you just have to present your argument well. Is it an attorney? More often than not, yes—and as knowledgeable and professional as that person is in his/her own field of expertise, the decision regarding your proposal may be based upon what that individual's experience was with a nurse the day they took their child to the Emergency Room. These are people, but they are not your colleagues. Approach them with respect and honesty, and state—in clear English, not in "nursese"—what it is you would like to do. This is neither the time nor the place for jargon or academic puffery. It is the time to frame your work within the perspective of the goals of your institution, and it is the place to bare your deep commitment and enthusiasm for what you hope to achieve through this project. If you are truly excited about what you are doing and committed to carrying the project through to a successful completion, that will be evident in your conversation and in your writing. If a foundation trusts you and finds your project feasible, and if your projected outcomes will forward the goals of the founders and trustees, you have a high probability of being funded.

By now, you have an appropriate funding source in mind, and you have spoken with someone at that source who has assured that your proposal is welcome, and you have the blessings (clearance) of your dean and development office to submit a proposal. In anticipation of this, you have reread the application guidelines and gathered the required proof of your school's not-for-profit status, board list, and budget (your financial or development office will have these documents). Meanwhile, you should also have been collecting your program data, plus letters of support from others sympathetic to your concept, plus an Institutional Commitment Letter from your dean—and from the external entities, if you are entering a new partnership. Text will also be needed to describe your own institution, and for this you may be wise to borrow approved "boilerplate" text from the school's public affairs office. In the concept paper, you already projected a total budget amount and committed to a goal and objectives. Half of the work is now done, and all you have to do is fill in the blanks. The structure of the proposal should follow the foundation's Application Guidelines to the letter. A formal Call for Proposals will include the preferred format, and it is not unusual today for a foundation to post its Call for Proposal and Application Guidelines on the Web (if instructions on the Web differ from the foundation's printed materials or letters, call to ask for clarification). Never be afraid of calling the program officer or their support staff when you have a legitimate question. Each contact with the funding source is another step in cultivation—that is, a way of getting to know each other.

You are now ready to go to work on the full proposal. As you approach the blank "piece of paper" on your computer screen, put yourself into the shoes of the program officer and the board of trustees. You know your project intimately, but they are coming to it cold. What's more, because they have so many proposals to read, you need to grab their attention within the first paragraph and compel them to read beyond page two. One's natural inclination is to list basic answers to who-what-why-how-and-where questions about a project, but that gets boring in a hurry. If a program officer is looking for projects to promote specific aspirations of the foundation, that officer is going to be more concerned about the outcomes you are expecting and how much money it is going to take to get there. It is best to encapsulate the scope of your project in an Executive Summary as an introduction to your proposal. Your first sentence should be the "ask," so that it is clear up front how much money you want for your project. This is not the time to be shy in talking about money. If you truly need and can justify the amount you are requesting, and if the homework you conducted has already revealed that this is an appropriate amount for that funder, have no fear. In that same sentence, include the full name of the institution that will receive the check, and the full name of the foundation from which you are requesting the grant—as well as the name of the particular funding initiative or Call for Proposals to which you are responding. Follow that with the title you have created for your program and a concise description of what could be achieved if you received funding (consider what you would like to see in the news headlines or in the annual report grant award briefs). If there are institutional partners involved, this is the time to name them (use each institution's official full name) and briefly state their role. Also, identify the proposed grant period, and if this is part of a larger project or program, help the funder to see how the pieces fit together. Close this paragraph with assurance to the funder that this project coincides with, and will help to promote, the mission and goals of your institution.

A question commonly heard from program officers today is, "What would happen if you did not do this?" Your next paragraph should offer text to describe and quantify the need for your project and proclaim its urgency. This is where you put to use the facts and statistics that you have already gathered. If the foundation has written substantially on the subject, refrain from telling them what they already know. But do relate those facts to your current situation, and when possible, include a trend chart or graph within the text to give a visual image of the history of the problem and the impact you hope to make (check the funder's guidelines to see if there is a limitation on attachments). Maintain a focus on the needs description by noting how your concept meshes with the mission of the funding source as well as with the goals of your institution (e.g., your strategic plan).

Now, in one or two sentences, state your overall goal, and follow that with a short list of specific measurable objectives. A common error is to promise too much for the size of grant being offered. Limit the number of objectives to what can actually be accomplished with the proposed size of grant, as later in the reporting process you will be held accountable for each item. Follow the list with text to describe an implementation strategy—the work to be done in order to accomplish each objective. The methods or strategy should be accompanied by a timeline for accomplishing each objective. Foundation personnel usually are most concerned about outcomes, so describe the methods and strategies within the context of anticipated results, and add only the detail necessary to convey that you understand the task at hand. If evaluation is a significant component of the project, that should be one of the objectives; devote the space necessary to concisely describe the tools and strategies you plan to use. Some foundations conduct independent evaluations of projects, so this may prompt another question to the program officer.

Finally, provide firm footing for your request by establishing your institutional credibility and that of the faculty who will be engaged in the project. Because there is so much you could say about your own and your school's successes, keep focused by thinking how you can help the foundation to appreciate your ability to perform as promised. If the funding source previously awarded grants to your school or institution, acknowledge that and tell (if applicable) how your project will build on that investment. Describe the resources (personnel, technical, etc.) available to support the project, and highlight the capabilities of the senior personnel on this project and the expertise that you can draw from (curriculum vitae of key personnel are a standard inclusion as an attachment to the proposal). If any faculty members on the project have been published in professional journals or written books on the topic, this provides great credibility, and you should be sure to include references to that text (hopefully you already have shared a copy of such an article with the program officer in one of your introductory meetings). Define the depth of your commitment in terms of the bottom line—at the end of the day, what will be different that can be attributed to the generosity of this grant—for the target population and for your school and/or institution.

The Budget and Justification are attached to the proposal narrative; the last paragraph of your proposal narrative should thus refer to those attachments. Summarize the size of grant requested, the anticipated grant/project period, and a brief recap of the expected impact. Just as in the preceding paragraphs, it is important to put life into this text. Of great importance to foundations today is the issue of sustainability, and this is the place to describe, if you have not done so already, what the legacy will be of your project once the grant funding has ended. If it is a community-based project, what equipment (if any) will be left with the community, and how will they know how to use it? If you are using a population to collect public health data, how will that community benefit from your work? If it is a successful demonstration project, how do you hope that it will be absorbed into existing institutions or practices? If this is to be an ongoing project, note how you will use this grant to leverage the interest of other funders. Again, reiterate the message from your Executive Summary regarding the bigger picture into which this project fits. This segues nicely into the level of significance this grant would have for your school as well as for the funding institution. Finally, promise that materials produced with the grant monies, or any publicity resulting from this grant, will acknowledge the funder.

The attached Budget and Justification must be an accurate reflection of the text in the proposal, and should relate directly to the objectives, methods and timeline. Be aware of your institution's policies and guidelines (e.g., percentage used for "fringe" benefits), and also learn what is acceptable to the funding institution (e.g., some foundations are skeptical of proposals that are top heavy with administrative costs; others don't fund equipment; also, most private foundations do not pay indirect costs—be sure to ask if the guidelines are not clear on these issues). The format of the Justification follows the format of the Budget. Be realistic about what and who is needed to achieve the objectives in the proposal, and in the Justification, clearly state how you arrived at the projected costs. In some very large foundations, the Justification is read separately from the proposal narrative (again, ask if you do not know), and when that is the case, be sure that the Justification narrative is thorough and compelling enough to stand on its own.

Finally, compile the proposal packet, and follow the foundation's guidelines for required attachments. Start with a simple one-page cover letter addressed to a specific person (with title) at the funding source, and if your submission is for a Call for Proposals, reference the name of the funding initiative to which you are responding. If your proposal packet is large, insert a table of contents (and double check to be sure the page numbers are correct). The proposal narrative will usually be followed by the Budget and Justification, proof of your institution's 501(c)(3) status, the resume of the principal investigator, and Letters of Support. Other attachments and appendices could include your school's operating budget and a list of the board of trustees (your institutional annual report may be the best way to provide this information), and charts and graphs to highlight need for your program (e.g., health indices of communities). It is helpful if the proposal narrative and budget/justification is printed with a "footer" showing your school's name, the funder's name, and the date of the proposal, along with the page numbers.

In some ways, the process is just starting; before you send the proposal to the foundation, it is important to submit your text to an internal review (many schools require a set amount of lead time to allow for this). The levels of review will vary from school to school, or from institution to institution, but start with the key persons who will be responsible for carrying out the program—those who had input and approval of your original concept paper, including the dean. If there are external partners in the program, they will get the next "pass." Finally, it will be most valuable if "your" program officer has time to give you an informal review and feedback. These people are very busy, but if they are aware of your program and want to fund it, they may be happy to make sure you have prepared a document to which the board will be receptive. At every step of the review process, be prepared to take the document back and rework the text. The finished product will be better for the extra effort.

Now the proposal has been submitted, and you have distributed copies to the key players on your project team so that they are fully knowledgeable in case someone calls from the foundation for information or further clarification. What can you do now? First and foremost, refrain from assuming you will get the grant, and do not under any circumstance list this funder as one of your supporters until you actually have the check in hand. If you mailed in the proposal (registered mail or a delivery service is advised), after a couple of days, call the foundation to make sure your proposal was received, and ask if they have questions. If the guidelines do not specify a timeline, it is fair to ask when the decision will be made. Do not be surprised if the foundation calls and asks you to rework the budget. Be gracious and do so, but also be cautious. If the revised amount is not sufficient to do what was proposed, that requires a discussion with the foundation. The worst case is that you will graciously decline the grant. The best case is that you and the foundation are able to work out a satisfactory compromise. The most difficult scenario is if the foundation requests that you find matching funds for a portion of what was requested, and that is the time to refer back to your file of other funders interested in this topic. Such a challenge may also appeal to some of your school's individual donors, so call in your development colleagues, dean, or trustees to make a presentation to selected individuals.

Your school's best opportunity to showcase all its capabilities, strong leadership, facilities, faculty, students, and programs is a Site Visit. When a foundation chooses to take the time to do this, such an opportunity can be a rewarding experience, although it requires planning and coordination. Talk with the foundation officer to determine exactly what they want to see, and ask if the trustees have a specific list of questions. Also determine how much time and leeway you have in planning the tour, and ask about the visitors' travel schedule. This is the time to pull out all the stops, so convene the faculty and administrative staff who are involved with the project and responsible for the advancement of the school, and plan an informational and inspirational tour. Fax an advance copy of the itinerary to the foundation, and include telephone numbers where their staff may contact them if needed. Welcome the foundation officers by picking them up at the airport or hotel (or invite them to join you for dinner the previous evening). Remember, these are important people, and they are also human; so if they are on a whirlwind tour of numerous sites, take cues from them throughout the day regarding their energy level, and build in breaks and telephone time as needed. You may want to begin the site visit with a brief overview of your school (a video is excellent to set the stage), and a round of introductions (know in advance who from the foundation will attend, and provide name badges). Give each participant a packet with the itinerary for the day (including the names and titles of all participants) as well as pertinent brochures or program information germane to their questions. To this packet, add a journal article or copies of publicity that your project has received. Plan into the schedule opportunities for the foundation representative to observe and talk with key faculty, and to have group interviews with (and/or demonstrations by) students. Do your best to rehearse these encounters in advance. You cannot "script" a student, but you can select your best representatives, emphasize the importance of what you hope to achieve, and help to instill confidence in the students so they are comfortable talking about their involvement with your project (the students can be the star attraction, and their comments are often the most remarkable segment of the site visit). If the project is a partnership, plan far enough ahead so that you can convene all of the leaders of the partner institutions (or advisory board) for a presentation and question-and-answer period with the foundation representatives (meet with this group in advance so they are fully informed about the site visit and what is expected of them). You will want to plan the seating for lunch, and use that time for directed conversation or for a presentation. It is important that you listen and watch carefully during the site visit to pick up on clues the foundation officer may convey. To be sure you have heard what you need to hear, end the tour with a summary of what has been on display that day, and use this opportunity to publicly thank all who participated—and to express your appreciation to foundation personnel for taking the time to come to visit. Follow this with a closed meeting for the foundation person to talk privately with the dean and a limited number of key players. This meeting is critical. Let the foundation person do the talking, and if follow-up is requested, do so within the week. Regardless of whether or not you get the grant at this point, you will know that you have done all you can to tell your school's story. If it is a good story, and if the experience has been genuine and informational, that will go a long way in solidifying a relationship for future grant opportunities.

Guess what: You got mail—and you're funded! Regardless of the size of the grant, an acknowledgement letter and official institutional receipt must be sent to the funder as soon as possible, especially from the dean or executive of your institution, and also from the president, if it is a significant grant. Often, a duplicate copy of the Award Letter will require the signature of the dean or financial executive of your institution before the check is mailed. If the check does not arrive until later, use that as an opportunity for the principal investigator to send a thank-you letter, and assure the grantor that you look forward to reporting on the outcomes that are achieved, thanks to their generous grant. Then check and double-check the due dates for those reports (progress narratives and financial reports sometimes have different due dates), and alert all who will be involved with you in preparing those reports. As you do the work of the project, pay attention to how you can quantify program impact to report back to the foundation. Also, jot down comments from participants or partners that might be included as testimonials in the report. If community advisory boards have been formed to assist with the project, track their meetings and participation. Many foundations like their grantees to share "lessons learned" so that others can gain from the process, as well. Be prepared to describe those lessons, as well as any changes that had to be made in order to meet the project objectives. Throughout the grant period, whenever publicity or program materials are published, be careful to include the name of the funder in print (again, check with the funding source if you have questions or if they require prior approval for use of their name), and include copies with your reports. Most of all, write a report that conveys the same enthusiasm and commitment for the project that you had in your original proposal. Each report is the next step toward your next grant.

In summary, successful grantsmanship is dependent first and foremost upon a precise fit of your concept with the goals and purpose of the funding body, and your presentation of a compelling argument to attract support for your project. Equally important is your ability to deliver on what was promised so that, as a good "steward" of the funder's investment, you can report positive and sustainable outcomes, and leverage that to further your vision. Your fundability will be enhanced measurably by the attention you continue to pay to building relationships, both internally among faculty, and externally with partners and with funding entities. Foundation and corporate development demands the best of cultivation and stewardship, and those efforts will be well rewarded.

REFERENCES

AAFRC Press Release. (1999, May 25). *Total giving increased 10.7% in 1998.* http://www.aafrc.org

9

Volunteers and Committees for Fundraising

Joyce J. Fitzpatrick and Sandra S. Deller

Volunteers are a very significant resource in fundraising; they can be asked to assist with a range of activities and can lead you to many other volunteers. Individuals can be asked to serve in many different roles, including chair or member of a committee, general advisor, or solicitor of peers. They can be instrumental in cultivation activities, such as hosting events or arranging key appointments, and most especially, they provide visibility to the school or institution in their circle of influence.

Volunteers both extend the fundraising capability of the development staff and executive, and also require a substantial amount of time from the staff. It is important to fully understand the various requirements needed for successful volunteer activities. The worst thing for any fundraising project is to have volunteers who are disillusioned because they do not view the successful outcomes that were promised in the introduction to the project. Remember that everyone wants to be part of a successful fundraising activity; everyone loves a winning team.

It is important to have a face-to-face conversation with each volunteer to request his/her participation. This is not only a courtesy, but also serves to orient the volunteer to the role that they are expected to assume and responsibilities inherent in the role. At this initial meeting the following topics should be discussed:

1. Overview of the school or institution, including mission, goals, and basic facts, for example, year of founding, number of alumni, students

and faculty; amount/number of research grants; a fact sheet with some comparative statistics demonstrating success is helpful;

2. Current development goals, including specific campaign goals if a campaign is planned or in progress;
3. Initial plans for achieving development goals;
4. Structure of campaign, including roles and responsibilities of professional development staff, committee structure, and general expectations of volunteers;
5. Specific expectations of each volunteer, including expected time commitment and level of personal or corporate gift expected/desired;
6. A list of other volunteers that you have recruited or hope to recruit;
7. Any benefits or rewards of supporting the institution.

While each development project or campaign will have specific needs, and thus, require certain kinds of volunteers, the following examples might be useful to consider: (a) volunteers who have influence, including community leaders and key foundation staff; (b) volunteers who have affluence, including philanthropists and CEOs of major corporations; and (c) volunteers who have connections, including alumni board presidents or past presidents. It is often considered that volunteers should contribute one of the three "W's" for fundraising purposes: work, wealth, or wisdom. Of course, volunteers who contribute more than one of these valuable resources are especially prized as members of any development committee or advisors in any way to the fundraising activities of the school or institution.

Each volunteer should be carefully selected considering the time, talents, and energy he/she can bring to the project. With careful preplanning and matching of volunteers to development goals and activities, there will be greater likelihood of success and a greater sense of fulfillment and satisfaction for the volunteer.

Throughout the campaign or agreed-upon length of commitment of volunteer, communication between professional staff and volunteers must be frequent, direct, personal, and sensitive. Each volunteer should receive regular phone calls from the development staff to make certain that the volunteer is up to date on important projects within the school or institution. Apprise them of recent accomplishments or successes. They should truly feel part of the "family," and they should know about key activities before they are more widely known. The volunteers should be treated as "insiders," made to feel as if they have the latest information about the school or institution, and that they receive the information before others.

All volunteers working with development staff should be treated with the utmost respect for their time and talents. Everyone is busy, and as we ask others to volunteer their time to our cause, staff support is critical. For example, never be late for a meeting with a volunteer; rather, value their time as a gift given to the campaign. Always return phone calls promptly from volunteers; they are your connections to funding. Define the goals and tasks for each meeting and interaction with volunteers, so that they are fully informed of your expectations. Always strive to place them in as positive a position as possible; and give them extra credit for everything that they do to assist with the fundraising. The more you nurture their contributions, including their time, talents, and resources, the more those contributions will grow.

COMMITTEES FOR FUNDRAISING

Committees should serve a purpose, and their work should be closely tied to the development goals. The individuals who are being asked to participate on committees are very busy and will want to know that their participation on a committee will be beneficial. During an active campaign, the development committee structure will be more elaborate than the committee structure for ongoing development activities. Even with beginning fundraising activities, there should, at the minimum, be an advisory board. If the fundraising effort will begin with the alumni fundraising around an annual fund goal, this advisory board can include primarily alumni of the school. If there are other donors that have already been identified, however, it would be good to ask them to also join the advisory committee.

The advisory committee can assist with overall assessment of the organization and realistic goal setting for fundraising for identified periods of time. These "insiders from the outside" will help you to answer the questions that will be raised by potential donors. In fact, they will give you an opportunity to anticipate some of the questions and objections that will be raised by others who are less familiar with the school or institution. At times, for example, alumni forget that the cost of tuition has increased considerably over the past two decades, and may not understand that the majority of students need some financial assistance. By asking the right questions early on in the planning stages, these volunteers may help you design your fundraising literature to address issues that would commonly be raised by alumni less familiar with the school. They can help you develop your "case statement" for your fundraising activities, and phrase the statement in ways that are easily understandable by potential donors.

While these committee volunteers will serve many functions for the school, it is important to keep the fundraising central to all discussions. The volunteers must be reminded that you want them to help achieve the goal, and that they can best assist you by providing contacts to potential funders.

When there is a formal campaign in progress, there is a need for more volunteers and for a more extensive committee organization. Generally, the larger the campaign goal, the more volunteers you will need. But even with a mini-campaign, it helps to have a formal committee structure. First of all, it makes it possible to involve more volunteers and to meet with committee members in a group. Secondly, you can develop specific goals for each of the subcommittees. The following are some suggestions for committee structures for a campaign:

Annual Fund Committee

Generally, the annual fund is supported by those constituents who are the closest to the institution. In the school of nursing, for example, the alumni make up the majority of the donors for the annual fund. This committee then, would consist of a chair who has been a major donor to the annual fund during previous years, and who has a commitment to the annual fund as a means of generating support.

Alumni Committee

Of course, this committee would only be relevant to schools of nursing or health science schools, not to health care institutions per se. It would consist of the most enthusiastic alumni, and those with influence who can encourage others to become involved. The chair should be an alumnus who is well known for previous involvement, one who is enthusiastic about the school and its goals for fundraising. This individual should be someone who has already made a major gift, a commitment for a major gift, or who has immediate potential to make a major gift.

Major Gifts Committee

This committee becomes very important in any campaign, as the majority of the funds will be raised from a small number of individuals. The committee should consist of individuals who have made major gifts or who have the potential to make major gifts, and who are inclined to do so in the current campaign.

Corporate Committee

This committee would consist of corporate executives who have some connection to the institution, either personally or through their business. In the case of a school of nursing, for example, the corporate committee could include individuals whose children or family have been students at the school. In forming the corporate committee, it is very helpful to know the institution's constituents at the local and national and, now, even at the international level. Corporate committee members can include those who have major health care businesses that are headquartered in the community or that have a significant business in the community served.

Foundation Committee

All foundations have individual participants who make decisions about how the money will be distributed. This often includes paid staff, program officers of foundations, and volunteers who may serve as members of distribution committees. The Foundation Committee should consist of persons who have foundation ties and relationships that would not present a conflict of interest in achieving the fundraising goals of the institution.

Campaign Committee

The Campaign Committee would consist of the chairs of the above-named committees. This overall committee would help coordinate the work of all other committees so that the fundraising potential is enhanced.

Goals of Committees

Prior to each meeting, the goals of each committee should be determined. In addition, the staff (development officer and dean or executive) should determine the percentage of the campaign goal that should be assigned to each committee. The staffing of each committee becomes the responsibility of the development officer in consultation with the dean or executive. Adequate staffing is critical to the success of involving volunteers, whether on an individual or committee level. No one likes to attend a poorly organized meeting; it is a waste of time and resources. For each meeting there should be a planned agenda, and a set of goals that the staff and committee chair want to accomplish in that specific meeting. For example, in the first meeting of the Major Gifts Committee, the goal could be twofold: to provide a comprehensive orientation to the committee members and, given the goals of the institution, to brainstorm about a list of possible major donors to the campaign. The members should also be engaged in rating of prospects for future gifts. The staff would follow up the meeting with individual contacts with each committee member to determine how each individual can best assist in either further identification of prospects or solicitation of potential donors.

Activities of Committees

Each committee should have an organized set of activities. A determination should be made about the activities necessary to achieve the desired campaign goals. The development staff should facilitate the accomplishment of the identified activities through consistent communication with committee chairs. Activities of the various committees can include the following examples: telethons for annual fund, special meetings to review prospect lists, and meetings to review goals and progress toward goals. Individual members of committees should be involved in solicitation of prospects, cultivation of donors, and recognition of contributors to their specific committee's goals.

THE DEVELOPMENT OFFICER'S PERSPECTIVE

Effective volunteers can be one of the development officer's most valued resources. It is important to consider their contribution in that context and treat them accordingly. First of all, conserve their time. This is the most precious commodity for all of us. Significant staff support needs to be allocated to managing, coordinating and communicating with volunteers. It is better to have fewer volunteers and treat them well.

Because of the significant time commitment, the selection of volunteers is critical. Identify and recruit only those volunteers who add value to the development effort. Each needs to be reviewed as carefully as you would in any hiring decision. Beyond defining their role and expected contribution, you need to have a clear understanding of their expectation of support. Each may vary slightly in their preferences or demands. This early dialogue can help to minimize any future difficulties.

Preparation for meetings with volunteers should be as thorough as prospect contact. After all, these can be your most significant donors. They need to always be presented in their role of representing your organization in the most favorable way. Their participation needs to be made as easy as possible by staff going the extra mile. Burn-out is not a phenomenon only applicable to staff. Ongoing feedback is critical to volunteer satisfaction and reinforces that they are in the loop.

Just like donors, volunteers can never be thanked too much. Make certain that they are recognized and given credit for any part played in a successful conclusion. The spotlight belongs to your volunteer. They are the true heroes. Do not let them be unsung heroes.

Volunteers have a network and talk to each other. If your organization has a good reputation in the use of volunteer talent, it will be easy to recruit and retain the type of leaders needed to meet your development objectives.

THE DEAN'S PERSPECTIVE

Health care institutions often rely on volunteers for many activities, and fundraising can benefit from executives' experiences with volunteers in other arenas. Volunteers often give of their time and talent because of the love of the cause. It is especially important to remember to nurture the volunteers, and praise their talents and contributions. Involve them as much as you can, without taking advantage of their time and talents. Keep the lines of communication open to them at all times. Remember, there should be no surprises to the volunteers, as they are to be embraced as team members. Because they join the team they move to a position of insider, and should be treated with respect and deference.

SUMMARY OF POTENTIAL CONTRIBUTIONS OF VOLUNTEERS

The key involvement of volunteers must, of course, be geared to the specific structure of the institution and its fundraising goals. The following list represents a summary of the many roles and responsibilities of volunteers in any fundraising effort. They include the following:

- Participate in designing the case statement;
- Review any written materials that may be used in the campaign;
- Help to identify fundraising goals;
- Identify other volunteers to serve in key roles;
- Identify potential sources of funds, including potential donors at the individual, foundation, and corporate level;
- Introduce the executive and development staff to new potential donors;

- Solicit donors with the dean/executive and/or development staff;
- Make a major gift to the campaign;
- Host receptions, events, meetings, and activities;
- Provide visibility to the institution through their participation;
- Serve as an ambassador for the institution;
- Keep dean and development staff aware of other community activities related to the fundraising of the institution;
- Help secure media coverage for key events of the institution; and
- Provide specific advice in their professional area of expertise, for example, financial planning, public relations, community organization of major benefits, and so on.

Although each volunteer should be selected for their individual strengths, there are certain characteristics that would be common to all volunteers. The following are key qualifications for any volunteer:

- Enthusiasm for the mission;
- Interest in people;
- Good interpersonal skills;
- Leadership skills;
- Broad-based contacts;
- Willingness to listen to others; and
- Organizational skills.

As with many other projects for the success of the campaign, the organization of the volunteer network is critical. Volunteers should feel as if they are central to the fundraising. They should be recognized and given credit at every opportunity. The development officer and dean should design the committees to build on the strengths of the individual volunteer participants and make every effort to give each of them sufficient activities to carry out to achieve campaign goals. The praise for volunteers and the recognition of their efforts should, however, exceed their involvement. That is, they should be given as high a profile as possible for their contributions, as this will often lead them to commit more time, energy, and resources in the future.

10

Campaigns

SANDRA S. DELLER AND JOYCE J. FITZPATRICK

Campaigns can provide major resources for an organization, and are most often the fundraising structure used to increase the number of major gifts for an institution. Campaigns also require unity of the institution's leadership and an intensive commitment of resources for a sustained number of years.

One of the earliest fundraising campaigns was that undertaken for Harvard College in 1641. In the 1820s, organized alumni and development activities were initiated by some leading educational institutions. It was not until the twentieth century that there was a focus on obtaining major gifts through fundraising activities. Campaigns provide a mechanism for focus on major gift fundraising.

The decision to mount a campaign is a serious commitment of time and resources on the part of any organization. To ensure success, there should be an established track record of effective, sustained fundraising. Consideration should be given to competition in the community. Are there other organizations or schools in your area already engaged in a campaign or planning a campaign? What are the possibilities of overlapping donors or priorities?

A campaign should be based on the institution's most significant priorities, not on a wish list of needs. These priorities must be defensible. They can be for capital needs, such as buildings or equipment, or for endowment, or for specific programmatic goals. Often, it comprises a mix of these fundraising priorities.

There can be a mini-campaign for a single facility or program initiative. Increasingly, institutions are in a continuous campaign mode. Annual funds are an important component of the campaign, and an effective campaign should increase yearly unrestricted gifts at the same time that multi-year restricted or endowment pledges are raised.

In the communication of a campaign to potential donors, the institution's case must be clearly described so that the donor believes it is worthy of support. A compelling rationale motivates donors to make major contributions.

Prior to initiating a significant campaign, it is advisable to retain professional fundraising counsel to do a feasibility study. This study tests the organization's potential ability to raise funds and the strength and influence of its various constituencies. The validity of the case and its appeal are measured. The assessment can serve as an indicator of the community's readiness to support such an effort. In the feasibility study, the relationship of key constituents to the institution and their interest and possible level of support are assessed. At the same time, all participants are educated on the institution's priorities through participation in the feasibility study. In an educational institution, input is sought from trustees, select groups of alumni, parents, business leaders, and foundation executives. The feasibility study may include a questionnaire and should have an individual confidential interview component with select individuals of influence or affluence. This process could also be accomplished by using a focus group led by a dean, trustee, or faculty member. However, objectivity is more difficult to achieve with an inside team. The interview or focus group should indicate a confidence level in the chief executive's ability to lead a successful campaign. The feasibility study will help formulate the goal and the timetable, and identify leadership or those capable of leadership gifts. Fundraising counsel can also recommend staffing patterns and an appropriate campaign budget.

The case for support, generally referred to as the campaign case statement, articulates the vision for the future and the institution's value to its community—locally, nationally, and globally. It is built on a long-range view of how an infusion of funds will better equip the institution to meet its mission now and in the future. The case statement should include gift opportunities and list the campaign leadership. Endorsements from influential constituents assist in validating the needs.

The authors participated in a campaign with an ambitious goal of raising $350 million over five years. Within the overall goal of $350 million, the university sought contributions in three areas:

- *Endowment*—Income from endowment enhances the quality of teaching, research, and scholarship. Significant increases in resources were needed to support education and research to attract and retain exceptional faculty in all fields.

- *Buildings and equipment*—In 1998, the university completed a master plan for the development of its 128-acre campus. The core of the plan revolved around the creation of a new center or heart for the campus: a library of the future and expanded student center.
- *Program support*—Support was sought for academic programs, services and other needed improvements throughout the university.

The motto chosen for the campaign for Case Western Reserve University was "A Convergence of Interests." With the Campaign goal a major issue, consultants were hired to test the feasibility of a $350-million target. They said that $300 to $325 million would be more realistic. The argument against a larger goal was more than a matter of subjective feelings. The external and internal infrastructure with which development professionals ordinarily begin a major campaign barely existed. With goals topping $1 billion at a few universities, campaigning in higher education has become a complex, specialized process. The traditional structure of volunteer committees working with professional staff is buttressed by meticulous research and planning and by sophisticated computer programs to assemble and analyze data on prospective donors.

Professionals begin a fundraising effort by constructing a pyramid of possible donors. A small number of possible top donors occupy the pyramid's peak; hundreds of prospects of more modest giving potential form the foundation of the pyramid.

The pyramid of donors referred to is the identification of a handful of potential mega-givers at the very top ($1 million plus), followed by major gift prospects ($100K to $500K). The next group is $25K to $100K. At the base are any donors up to $10K. It is typical to find many new prospects at the base. However in our case, we had not had an active development program until the president arrived in 1987, and therefore there was a paucity of identified prospects. With the clock ticking, we had to hit the road and visit, cultivate, and solicit prospects as quickly as possible.

As the Campaign progressed, the university built on the strong positive feelings of alumni by increasing and renewing ties with graduates through a host of new activities. Alumni with the potential to consider major gifts or to be helpful in the campaign were invited to attend President's Weekends on the CWRU campus.

The President's Weekends offered a select group of alumni and friends an "insider's view" of the university through personal contact with the president and his wife, star faculty, and students. During the campaign, this was a semiannual 2-day event, taking place in the spring and fall. The programs were designed to build enthusiasm for the present and future, and guests were asked to recall their memories or impressions of their days on campus. These events were enormously successful in accelerating the cultivation process for major gift prospects.

Other activities included the establishment of alumni chapters in cities with a critical mass of alumni. These activities provided an additional volunteer base and forum to host the president and promote the Campaign. During the Campaign period, the university established 16 regional alumni chapters: Boston, Chicago, Cincinnati, Columbus, Detroit, Houston, Los Angeles, New York City, Orange County (California), Philadelphia, Pittsburgh, San Diego, San Francisco, Miami, and Washington, DC.

At the time of the campaign, the University had more than 86,000 living alumni. Approximately two-thirds of the alumni lived outside of the Cleveland area. After Ohio, the second and third largest concentrations of CWRU alumni were in the states of California and, on the East Coast, in the tri-state area of New York, New Jersey, and Connecticut.

The National Campaign was divided into three regions: East Coast, West Coast, and Central—with campaigns in the cities of New York, Boston, Washington, D.C., San Francisco, Los Angeles, Akron, Columbus, Cincinnati, and Chicago. For the campaign, we established a physical presence in the East Coast, with an office, development director, and assistant in Washington, D.C. The West Coast office and staff were located in San Francisco. Prospects in Ohio and other Midwest cities, were covered from Cleveland.

The Campaign leadership comprised three prominent representatives to the national campaign advisory committee and two major executives selected from the Board of Trustees (all trustees were involved in some way.) Another main committee was the Major Gifts committee. It consisted of 17 members and two co-chairs. Ten at-large members constituted the core. The other seven members were representatives from the Campaign committees of each of the professional schools and the undergraduate colleges. Each member was to serve a 2-year term with the opportunity to be reappointed.

PUBLIC RELATIONS

Promotional material was developed to support the fundraising effort by presenting the case for support, highlights of past and present accomplishments, and future potential that the campaign vision would achieve. Endorsements of community leaders were prominently displayed. There was a specific brochure for the university, which provided an overview of the total campaign goals. The mechanisms for giving and giving opportunities were also discussed. Another brochure was developed for the corporate campaign by the public relations agency. Each school had a campaign brochure illustrating their discipline-specific needs; for example, the School of Nursing brochure was titled "New Dimensions in Nursing." It served both as a pride piece for our tradition of leadership in nursing education and articulated emerging priorities for education, research, scholarship, and practice. Like the university brochure, it listed the campaign leadership of all committees and the cost and rationale for campaign goals.

During the campaign, the university published quarterly reports or updates. Each of the schools used their newsletters to keep alumni and friends informed about the progress on goal attainment.

During the campaign we took every opportunity on a university-wide and individual school perspective to promote the campaign in stories about donors or any related campaign activities.

THE SCHOOL OF NURSING CAMPAIGN

The School of Nursing had a goal of $15 million. The silent phase, or advance fund, began in July of 1987. This is done to raise leadership gifts and commitments from the "insiders" of the institution. At announcement on December 31, 1989, we had a total of $5,416,000. This meant that we needed to raise approximately $599,000 a quarter over the length of the campaign; we hoped to conclude the campaign by December 31, 1993.

The task was made especially daunting because the Nursing School had just completed a campaign for $5.5 million for critical care nursing in June of 1987. We had been aggressive before, but had also been more regionally focused. If we were to meet the challenging campaign goals, we needed to raise funds from alumni all across the country.

We increased visibility of the School through informational pieces, newsletters, conferences, and special events. The dean, faculty, and development staff traveled nationally to cultivate and solicit prospects. When they were attending a conference or presenting a lecture, they combined academic affairs with development objectives whenever possible.

When time did not permit a personal visit, faculty contacted alumni by phone.

A solid structure for campaign activity was created through our campaign committee. Co-chairs for the School were a chief executive from a large health care corporation and a much beloved alumni leader. An alumni committee was created to identify local and regional alumni volunteers. The structure also included other select committees for targeted groups. The Corporate Committee led by the health care executive leader recruited other corporate leaders. There was a major gifts component and a special initiative for physicians. A Special Projects Committee focused on a special event to raise both visibility and funds.

The Corporate Committee was led by our co-chair, who was the health care executive. We targeted business leaders who had some connection to health care. This connection could be by virtue of their business relationship to health care, their philanthropy or, in some cases, because their wives, mothers, daughters, sons, or other loved ones were in the profession. We recruited members through individual meetings and held a series of power breakfasts on current issues in health care. The group was expanded by asking each to recruit two to three associates with a similar profile. They were each solicited and chose a short list to personally solicit with the dean and development officer.

The Major Gifts Committee was led by a recognized Clevelander and an alumna who was a trustee. Our co-chairs were also members. For the Nursing School campaign, we considered major gift prospects at $25,000 and above. The university defines major gifts at $100,000 and above. Prospects were selected. Specific strategies and call assignments were coordinated by the development office.

The Physician's Committee was chaired by a physician friend of the School who was a trustee. His daughter-in-law was an alumna of the Nursing School. The model was an emphasis on the physician-nurse collegial partnership. The strategy for recruiting members and process was the same as the Corporate Committee. The dean and development officer had individual follow-up meetings with members to enhance their cultivation before solicitation, to develop the relationship to the school and a commitment to its needs.

The Physician's Committee was given a boost when a prominent physician CEO made a commitment in honor of his wife who was a nurse. She was not herself a graduate of our school, but a volunteer member of the School's advisory committee and a good friend of the School.

The Special Projects Committee, led by a benefit expert, assembled a group of socialites and School supporters. The benefit was christened "Nightingala" and celebrated Florence Nightingale's birthday and the Bolton School's commitment to the community through the reinstitution of the Bachelor of Science in Nursing Program. This event was very successful and raised approximately $55,000 for the undergraduate program scholarship fund.

The Nursing Campaign secured gifts and commitments totaling $26.3 million surpassing our $15 million goal. The campaign attracted funding for three new endowed professorships in nursing, pediatrics, and oncology.

CAMPAIGN BUDGET

In the planning process, a budget for the campaign needs to be considered. Obvious costs include fundraising consultation for the feasibility study or a retainer for the consultant to review benchmarks for the campaign's progress. Even without using a consultant, there should be monies allocated for extra fundraising expenses. Additional professional or support staff may need to be recruited. A campaign coordinator can provide tracking of prospects and maintain current records and information flow. A research or research assistant might be another consideration. If constituents are located nationally, a travel budget should be a cost component. If national travel is not a consideration, funds should be allocated for increased cultivation expenses, such as breakfasts, lunches, dinners, or special events. Typical special events generally include a kick-off announcement and a campaign celebration or wrap-up. All include mementos or tribute tokens to thank volunteers.

Public relations/promotional materials, especially some illustrative brochures explaining the case, options for giving, and endorsements by community leaders should be budgeted. The elaborateness of the printed or promotional materials should be consistent with the goal's size and, most important, with the organization's image and constituent expectations. Sometimes a minimalist approach—a simple, quality piece, that is not ostentatious or too costly is preferred.

In preparing a budget, the staff and administration should consider all the various constituencies, as well as some unexpected expenses in developing a budget for review and endorsement by the board prior to the campaign. Fundraising cannot occur in a vacuum; there needs to be resource allocation up front. Realistic expectations before, during, and after campaigning are an integral component of the campaign.

CAMPAIGN WRAP-UP AND CELEBRATION

A successful campaign is reason to celebrate. It is an opportunity to give visibility to the organization and to acknowledge the contributions of volunteers and donors. Beyond this, it sets the stage for the next fundraising initiative or campaign.

For the university, we scheduled campaign wrap-up celebrations in cities with alumni chapters and regional campaign committees. The president or trustee was present, along with key members of the development staff. A brief video showcasing new buildings and highlights of new programs made possible by the campaign gave alumni a sense of ownership. There was a summary of gifts as a "report to shareholders." The festivities culminated in a Cleveland event for all $10,000-plus donors, including individuals, family foundations, corporate and foundation representatives, national campaign leadership, Cleveland campaign volunteer leadership, trustees, honorary trustees, deans, and administrators.

Campaign leadership volunteers received an engraved crystal "star" with the university seal. All major donors ($100,000 plus) also received the star. Donors at $10,000 and above were presented certificates—special calligraphy keepsakes in custom framing. Endowment fund donors received a copy of their endowment resolution approved by the Board of Trustees.

Each of the schools held a special recognition and celebration event. The School of Nursing recognized its donors in several ways. A glass wall hanging, etched with the names of all donors who gave major gifts to the campaign (over $10,000) was commissioned for the main lounge of the School of Nursing. A reception was held in the lounge to unveil the glass etched hanging. As expected, all of the donors gravitated towards the hanging, to view it and, undoubtedly, to determine if they were correctly represented. The wall hanging then served as a "talking point" for potential future donors.

A luncheon was held to celebrate the successful conclusion of the campaign, and to thank all of the major donors. At the invitation of the dean and development officer, one of the corporate executives, who had served as co-chair of the School of Nursing campaign committee, agreed to host the luncheon at his home. This was particularly important, as this businessman was a community leader. Thus, his active support of the School of Nursing served an important function in raising the over-all visibility of the School in the larger community.

DEVELOPMENT OFFICER'S PERSPECTIVE

The university campaign catapulted our fundraising to a new level. The return on this institutional investment continues to be strong. Private support has more than doubled since the campaign, with an endowment over $1.4 billion. The precedent for a significant level of fundraising has been set and is now an expectation, even without the momentum of a campaign.

In addition to the generation of many new funds, the campaign also led to an increased number of volunteers and donors joining the university leadership as trustees or members of key committees. A national presence in contacting alumni and friends has provided a large volume of prospects. Now the challenge is to sustain the national visibility and presence.

Individual sights have been raised by the campaign in the size of gifts and the types of capital projects that the university constituents are capable of supporting. A renewed appreciation and sense of pride has emerged. The campaign was the catalyst to unite alumni. Donors feel they are share-holders, and now often suggest other alumni who could be contacted now.

The School of Nursing enjoyed a similar experience in donor identification and prospect growth. The annual fund grew and prospered as a result of the campaign. Volunteer leadership continues to be an important resource for the school.

DEAN'S PERSPECTIVE

This major campaign for the School of Nursing made it possible to formalize a strategic plan that would be implemented over several years. As the case statement for the School's campaign was developed, so was the strategic plan, as it was believed that with such a significant goal, we had to have major projects to propose to donors.

In many ways, campaigns offer the catalyst for broad-based development activities. They also offer an opportunity to create structures around which you can formalize fundraising goals. The "excuse" of a campaign and a specific goal provides a platform on which to begin a discussion with all potential donors.

In summary, the university campaign far surpassed its goal, raising $416.5 million, and results continue to reverberate to the present. At the campaign's conclusion in 1994, 31 new endowed professorships were created and 102 new scholarships and fellowship funds established. An additional 65 endowed funds were created for financial aid and student loans. Endowment was increased substantially. A very significant fundraising yardstick, the annual private support, grew from $25.8 million 10 years previous to $77 million in 1994. Research rankings rose and numbers and quality of students gained significant increases.

ACKNOWLEDGMENT

Note: Information regarding the CWRU capital campaign was obtained from the CWRU magazine; permission to use this information was obtained from the editorial staff.

11

Stewardship and Recognition

SANDRA S. DELLER AND JOYCE J. FITZPATRICK

Stewardship is both the beginning and end of a solicitation program. If institutions gave their stewardship activities the priority that successful businesses give their customer relations activities, they would truly enjoy many happy returns.

Effective stewardship requires an integrated institutional commitment. In a university setting, for example, it could involve the president, provost, deans, faculty, development officers, alumni relations professionals, gift processing/accounting, and research personnel. A coordinated effort and team approach is desirable involving all areas related to donor acknowledgment. Appointing a stewardship or central contact person coordinator will help ensure an effective program. Usually the development officer responsible for the solicitation initiates the activity. The stewardship coordinator provides a safety net to make certain that all donors regardless of gift size are thanked.

When communicating with donors to acknowledge their gift, accuracy is the essential first step. There needs to be verification that the thank-you has the correct amount, that the name is spelled correctly, and that the preferred form of address is adhered to in the communication. The gift's purpose must also be represented correctly. Typical faux pas in gift reporting are sins of omission, such as failing to put the right number of "0's," or stating the purpose of the gift incorrectly, or conditions not agreed on by the donor. Any of the above could cause irreparable damage to the donor relationship, whether it is a new or previous donor. New donor relationships are particularly sensitive.

Donors should be treated with the same courtesy that we use in personal life. All of us remember procrastinating over a thank-you note to a relative. Timeliness is valued. The responsiveness of an organization to a donor's generosity should never be underestimated. Donors do notice, and often call if they have not received acknowledgments promptly. Older donors really appreciate this trait, as they are often more anxious about checks or monies sent.

The acknowledgment needs to fit the gift size. Donors do not expect to receive effusive acknowledgments for modest contributions. Letters or notes need to, first of all, be sincere. All contributors want to know that the gift is appreciated and how it will be used by the organization. For smaller gifts, the donor can be thanked for their participation or for remembering the institution again this year.

Following a successful solicitation, the donor should be immediately thanked. If more than one individual participated in the solicitation, ideally, they should all send a brief personal note of appreciation.

For major gifts, the donor and the gift should be acknowledged by the president and/or dean/chairperson. A cardinal rule is that a donor can never be thanked too much or too often. For significant donations, there might be a special memento given. This could be a replica of your institution's landmark building or its logo or most recognizable symbol. For example, a children's museum in the Midwest once commissioned a miniature locomotive as their major gift recognition piece for their campaign. Their train collection was one of its signature displays and the pride of that museum. The miniature locomotives quickly became a status symbol among that city's corporate elite.

If there has been a family history of philanthropy, an album could be produced that would feature the participants and their legacy through the years. For donors to capital projects, a collage could depict the stages of construction, from groundbreaking through building dedication.

Some institutions create a special society or membership for high-end contributors. These VIPs might be designated by a special association name and a unique symbol created to identify the wearer as a privileged member. Such an association should have some attendant benefits, such as a special event annually acknowledging this group and its influence. This helps to reinforce how much the institution values their support and friendship. Such special attention promotes additional gifting. These are also the individuals who should be personally called, e-mailed, or faxed with any priority institutional news. They need to be treated as part of the inner circle with frequent communication.

For some of these very significant donors, there could be a photo and a brief profile included in the institutional Web site. Creating a special society or name for these major donors is challenging. Some institutions prefer to celebrate their legacy by adopting the name of well-known historical leader of the institution. For institutions with a distinctive building or campus landmark, this might inspire the name or symbol. Geography, too, can help identify constituents, if this is relevant, especially with alumni chapters or clubs in other cities. There are also more general designations for lifetime donors. At Case Western Reserve University, the Society of ENDOWMENTORS is a special organization for individuals who have made any kind of endowment or planned gift. The Möbius strip, with its unending surface, symbolizes the perpetuity of the gifts to endowment.

Young alumni are an important donor constituency and a special organization created for them could sustain their loyalty. Activities and all communications with these younger donors require tailoring to their needs and style. Research indicates that younger people want more of a sense of partnership in their gifting. They desire accountability of how their gifts are used, and for what purpose, and expect to see results. Unlike some of their fathers, mothers, grandmothers, and grandfathers, these donors will not give out of a sense of philanthropy or habit, but rather to accomplish something important. Some institutions are recognizing cumulative giving to promote a pattern of philanthropy. For example, recognitions have been developed for multiyear total giving.

In the well-publicized "transfer of wealth," women are controlling and will control significant resources—and not just inherited wealth; much of it will be money they have earned themselves. Women respond differently as donors than do men. They tend to be more innovative, and may support organizations that they perceive are making a difference in causes they value. Like younger donors, they too are result-oriented and seek a partnership. They are informed givers; therefore, it is essential that stewardship be responsive to their desire for communication. When possible, their input should be sought on their philanthropy.

As with all aspects of individual fundraising, stewardship should be tailored as much as possible to the individual. Focused activities and recognition are the ties that bind to the institution.

All donors deserve recognition. It is helpful to publish a list of all donors in some printed material. It could be a special recognition piece or insert in another publication. Donors like to see their name in print. If there are categories of gifting, this can encourage people to stretch to the next level. Peer pressure or desire to be on the same list with a "mover and shaker" can be a strong motivator. Aside from the donative factor, it is helpful to demonstrate to others in the community the breadth and level of your supporters. An Annual Report is another good mechanism for listing your donors. Whatever method you choose to publish donor names, make certain that someone who has a good institutional history, and is familiar with many of the donors, proofs the list for accuracy, paying special attention to individuals who are divorced or to married women who prefer to use their maiden or professional name. Additionally, deceased donors could be listed, with that status duly noted, as well as any anonymous gift, if designated for a specific purpose. Gift levels must be correctly categorized.

Recognition always raises the issue of how gifts are counted. Is it by calendar or fiscal year? Annual funds need to be counted according to the deadline for the Annual Fund Campaign. How matching gifts are handled is equally important. If donors can advance their gift level with their company's participation, it will maximize their contribution and motivate them to apply for the matching gift—a win-win for the donor and institution.

Most couples expect to have their gifts counted together. However, some spouses have such a strong individual identity that they prefer to be recognized individually. Another consideration is lifetime giving or cumulative gifting. Some institutions have special categories for individuals who have achieved a six-figure gift over a lifetime of institutional giving. The national organization dedicated to fundraising, the Counsel for Advancement and Support of Education (CASE), has guidelines for gift counting. (See Appendix B for more information regarding CASE.)

Someone has to be responsible for coordinating the logging of gifts and the mailing of receipts for income tax purposes. It is essential that receipts, like acknowledgments, be sent as soon as possible. Nothing can discourage additional donations more than tardy acknowledgments. Donors should never have to call to request their receipts. It might be desirable to institute a policy of sending the thank-you and receipt within a week of the gift's receipt.

If there are premiums or tokens attached to membership categories, someone needs to be assigned responsibility for the packaging and shipping of these items. In planning donor gift items, there should be an awareness that the Internal Revenue Service imposes certain limits for gifts or appreciation memorabilia given to donors in return for their donation. If premiums exceed this amount, the donors may have to subtract the cost of the token from their charitable donation.

Another critical aspect of stewardship is a report to the donors on the use of their gift, particularly important for donors to endowment funds. How often they receive a report depends upon the resources of the institution. At least once per year donors should receive information indicating the market value of their fund, including interest earned. A description of the allocation of the fund will encourage satisfaction with their investment. For scholarship funds the number of students supported and the amount of each student's support should be reported. Donors for faculty development should receive a report of faculty accomplishments or activities. Donors to professorships should be kept abreast on an ongoing basis of recent research publications, lectures, or programs involving their chair-holders. If donors have participated in a campaign, they should receive an update on the campaign progress or successful conclusion, again, relating this to their gift whether it was for capital improvements or endowment. Even donors to annual funds like to hear about reaching the goal and what this will enable the institution to accomplish.

Special events can enhance stewardship. Donors to scholarship funds could be invited to a breakfast or brunch to meet their scholars. The format could include an address by a scholarship donor and an impressive student recipient. At the very least, student scholars should be encouraged to write a letter or note to their donor, personally thanking them for their support. The letter can include information about how they selected their school (program), future plans, and the importance to the scholar and/or their family of the scholarship assistance. If possible, a meeting of donor and scholar reinforces the donor's satisfaction, and could, in some cases, provide valuable contacts for the student.

For donors to professorships, there might be a special event created to spotlight this select donor constituency. When possible, donors should be invited to meet their chair-holders. If a special event or meeting is difficult to arrange, donors should be invited to attend an address or conference presented by their endowed professor.

The authors are most familiar with a special stewardship program. This ensures that each school's development officer prepares an annual letter to each donor or family member of an endowment fund reporting on how their funds are benefiting that particular school. Quarterly tickler reports are sent to the development officer to remind them to prepare and send their stewardship letters detailing the market value and endowment's purpose. They are encouraged to draft a personalized stewardship letter for their dean and send it to the donor.

It may be helpful to survey key institutions in your area to determine what stewardship activities they employ, especially for major donors. While it is always desirable to initiate a program unique to your institution, it is helpful to learn how other institutions manage donor relationships. There might be an opportunity to adapt another institution's successful technique.

An effective stewardship program can increase revenues. Through tracking and contact with the donors of established endowment funds, there may be an opportunity to raise the level of the fund, for example, from a financial assistance fund (approximately $20,000) to a full scholarship fund (approximately $200,000), or a visiting professorship (approximately $500,000) to a full professorship (approximately $1,500,000). (Note that these amounts cited here may vary from institution to institution.) Future solicitation is supported by timely and thorough annual stewardship reporting.

DEVELOPMENT OFFICER'S PERSPECTIVE

As rudimentary as it sounds, treat your donors with the same respect you would treat friends. Friends require ongoing communication and time. These donors are your institutional friends; they will remember if they have been treated well or suffered from benign neglect.

In our scurrying to secure more and larger gifts, it is a challenge to remember those who have contributed, but perhaps on a smaller scale. These donors may surprise you. Some may have been unable to make another gift to a fund, but feel sufficiently good about their investment that they will reward the organization in their will.

DEAN'S PERSPECTIVE

Every donor is valuable to the institution. It is important to treat current students as potential alumni donors, and current small gift donors as potential major gift donors. The most important aspect of stewardship and recognition is communication. It is important to keep in mind that, generally speaking, the more personal and direct the communication, the better. Also, in most cases, donors like more communication and contact, rather than less.

12

Case Studies

JOYCE J. FITZPATRICK AND SANDRA S. DELLER

Based on our many years of experience in fundraising, we could identify several case studies to illustrate the various aspects of fundraising that we have included in this book. We have chosen a few examples that we believe are most illustrative of the common experiences that are encountered in fundraising.

CASE STUDY #1: AN ALUMNI GIFT INCREASED OVER TIME AND INVOLVEMENT

Dr. CC, an alumna of the School of Nursing from the 1940s, retired from an exciting professional career in nursing. Along with her husband, a public health professional and faculty member at a large Midwestern university, CC traveled and consulted extensively for the World Health Organization. She was not known to the school as a potential major donor until the "wrap-up" phase of an early campaign, one for $5.5 million dollars, that was successfully completed. At the end of this campaign, a letter was sent to all alumnae, notifying them that the campaign would be ending, and asking if they would like to contribute. CC identified herself as a major donor, indicating that she would like to give away vacation property that she and her husband had bought for retirement purposes. Her husband had recently died and she did not wish to maintain the property alone. The university accepted the property, which, when sold, amounted to a gift of approximately $150,000. This was the beginning of a significant relationship with this alumna which lasted several years.

As key representatives of the school, we brought CC into many new networks with us. She joined the Visiting Committee, a group of influential persons whose responsibility it was to advise the dean. We also asked her advice and opinion about several of our programs, including those of particular interest to her based on her professional background. At the time of her initial gift, the School had little involvement in the international nursing community. But as the years passed, the mission of the School changed, and became more focused on global nursing.

Because CC had an extensive involvement in international work, we invited her to join us in traveling to international conferences and workshops. Twice she accompanied faculty to Italy. Over a period of approximately 10 years, we built a strong relationship with this donor. She made it clear that she did not want personal recognition for her gifts. She wanted to be helpful behind the scenes, particularly if there were any special needs of students.

As CC's involvement with the School grew, so did the size of her gift, to one of several hundred thousand dollars. Eventually the School was named as the major beneficiary of her estate, because she had no family heirs and no other major interests.

How did this gift occur? CC reached out to the School at a time in her life when she was very alone, and we responded to her need for involvement with a worthwhile project. She was especially eager to relate to students and faculty who benefited from her many small gifts over the years. She liked the personal contact, the friendship, and the camaraderie that accompanied her gift.

CASE STUDY #2: A GRATEFUL PATIENT'S SPOUSE

Mr. J was a "self-made" millionaire, having been successful with several different investments early in his business career. He and his wife, M, had no children. Early in the marriage, M was diagnosed with multiple sclerosis. For several years she lived with the illness. Mr. J was devoted to his wife, and made certain that she received the best care possible. Throughout her life she had several peak periods of illness; often she was hospitalized during these acute episodes. Her illness progressed to the point where it was necessary to have 24-hour care provided for her in the home. Mr. J hired private nurses for this care. Throughout M's illness, Mr. J knew that it was the quality of the care provided by the nurses that made a difference in M's quality of life with multiple sclerosis.

Mr. J committed funds in support of nursing education so as to better prepare future generations of nurses to care for patients like his wife. In total, millions of dollars of support have been provided over the years to individual nurses, through fellowships offered through the foundation Mr. J established, and to endowment funds at two schools of nursing. Following Mr. J's death, the foundation support continued to be channeled into health care. In addition to the support provided to nursing education, Mr. J's foundation also provided support for the establishment of a multiple sclerosis center at one of the leading local health care institutions. Mr. J restricted his support to funding of projects in the community where he and his wife lived for all of their adult life. Because he made his fortune in that community, he wanted to give back to that same community.

It is not only the story of Mr. J that is significant here, although his commitment to nursing education was great. But even after his death, the foundation he established continues to support nursing. In fact, the head of the foundation committed substantially more funds to the School of Nursing after Mr. J's death. Mr. F, a friend of Mr. J, thought that something should be done to boost the quality of clinical nurses prepared for health care delivery. He offered the School a $2 million challenge grant that led to a mini-campaign for acute and critical care nursing. Through this campaign, an additional $3.5 million was raised. On the recommendation of Mr. F, the majority of the money was committed to a professorship, which is named in honor of both Mr. and Mrs. J.

CASE STUDY #3: A GIFT OF RECOGNITION FROM THE HUSBAND OF AN ALUMNA

The Smiths lived on the East Coast and had a large family and ties to Dr. Smith's school. Mrs. S had been a friend of the school for years and was a steady donor. She had been giving $1000 annually since 1982. Former development officers and deans had done a good job of cultivating her and developing the relationship through calls, letters, and occasional visits. Mrs. S' husband was an Ivy League alumnus, a physician and entrepreneur. Dr. S was a major donor to his alma mater, and when we were introduced to him, Dr. S was assisting his school with raising thousands of dollars for its annual fund.

The couple had strong roots in Cleveland. Dr. S had a brother who was a dual graduate of the College of Arts and Sciences and the Law

School. Another brother had attended the College of Arts and Sciences. Their sister worked at the University, and her husband was also a graduate.

The dean had introduced our new university president to Dr. and Mrs. S, and a good dialogue had begun. The dean had relatively frequent professional conferences in the area where the Smiths lived; she would use that occasion to further the cultivation through lunches and dinners.

During one of these visits, the dean introduced to Dr. S the concept of doing something significant to honor Mrs. S at her nursing school. While initially he appeared to like the idea, he was not overly enthusiastic. The university and the school were in a campaign. Thus, we needed a persuasive reason to have Dr. S. make his ultimate gift to the Nursing School for his wife during the campaign.

In the spring of the following year, Mrs. S would celebrate her 60th alumni reunion. This would become our rationale. A trustee who was from a distinguished family, and knew Dr. and Mrs. S, offered to assist in the solicitation. The president, dean, and trustee flew to the east coast to meet with Dr and Mrs. S.

During the meeting the dean proposed the 60th reunion as an occasion to honor Mrs. S by establishing a professorship in her honor. The dean appealed to his fundraising knowledge and expertise, as well as his understanding of the example this would set for other nursing graduates. Also, he was aware of how significant such a gift would be to the school at this time, both nationally and internationally. Through his long career, Dr. S had always respected and valued nurses; he clearly recognized their contributions. Dr. S liked the concept, and agreed to give it serious consideration. Essentially, the gift was made. All that remained was to work out the funding. It was funded through a combination of outright and planned gifts.

The S' endowment gift of close to $2 million was the largest gift to the school during this campaign. Mrs. S had been a public health nurse and a devoted mother. She had worked to put Dr. S through school, and they were truly partners in his many successful endeavors. The dean had proposed pediatrics as the possible focus area of the professorship, and they immediately warmed to the concept. This was to be the first professorship in the world in Pediatric Nursing. This would enable the school to attract a renowned scholar to the school.

The trustee who had participated in the solicitation hosted a gala reception to mark this milestone for nursing and the school.

Why did Dr. and Mrs. S decide to make this gift? The 60th anniversary was certainly not that compelling a reason. We had done a good job of building the relationship and involving Mrs. S in the school's programs and plans for the future. Dr. S wanted to demonstrate his appreciation to his wife for her indefatigable support. As a savvy fundraiser, he knew the value of such a gift to raise the sights of other donors. The timing was right, but the seeds had been planted many years before.

13

Staffing the Development Office and Other Organizational Issues

JOYCE J. FITZPATRICK AND SANDRA S. DELLER

The staffing of the fundraising activities for any organization is an important component for the dean or executive to consider. A good staff and organization will contribute substantially to helping achieve the goals for fundraising. In our experience in consulting with other schools of nursing and health care organizations in the initial stages of launching fundraising activities, this is one of the most overlooked areas. Sometimes, the belief exists that "anyone can do fundraising." Therefore, professional development help is not thought to be needed. Another major misperception is that "If the programs are excellent, donors will want to give us their support."

STAFFING THE DEVELOPMENT OFFICE

Professional development staff should be employed for the fundraising activity. There are a number of ways to identify development professional candidates for employment once the needs of the organization have been assessed and the position description developed. Often, development professionals know each other in the community, and a one-to-one referral can be made. Other resources that might be helpful are the program officers at local foundations, and the local or regional branches of the major organizations for fundraising staff. It may be helpful to look at the second-in-charge at a competing institution; a position as director of development may offer an opportunity for career advancement that would not be available for some time in their current place of employment.

Even if the institution can only afford a part-time individual, it is important to have a professional fundraiser in the position. If it is impossible to hire even a part-time individual, perhaps there is someone in the community who has retired from a professional fundraising position who would be willing to provide one day/week as a volunteer. But even this becomes problematic, as the internal structures and the follow-up for any fundraising activity are two of the most overlooked and most critical elements. All good intentions and plans can be inconsequential if there is not prompt follow-up with prospects. The plan for follow-up and overall organization of the fundraising activity is the responsibility of the development professional in consultation with the executive.

In a major campaign, the development office may be staffed with several individuals, each with very specific responsibilities. For example, in planning for a multimillion-dollar campaign, it would be helpful to have one staff member responsible for overall development activities, with two assistants: one with responsibility for alumni and annual fund activities, and the other with responsibility for foundation and corporate fundraising. Clerical and support staff members also are necessary.

One of the members of the development staff office should be extremely conscientious regarding details. There need to be adequate systems for research on potential donors, for filing reports, and for project description and tracking. The executive should never meet with a potential or current donor without having all the prospect information available that is relevant to the solicitation. There must be mechanisms created to brief the executive before meetings, and methods for summarizing the results of every meeting with donors and volunteers. The more organized the development office, the more likely you will be successful in fundraising.

The executive should hire the professional fundraiser because he or she is the person with whom the fundraiser will have the most direct and consistent contact. It is imperative that the executive and professional development officer have a very close working relationship, and that they understand that, to be successful, their roles must complement each other. It goes without saying that there should be no competition between the executive and the development officer. The development officer must understand his or her role in supporting the institution and, therefore, in supporting the executive.

INTERNAL STRUCTURES FOR DEVELOPMENT

No matter how many staff members are in the fundraising office within the organization, there should be an understanding of the value, purpose, and goals of fundraising among staff at all levels of the organization. In other words, it is important for the executive to clearly articulate that fundraising is an integral component of the work of the organization. The fundraising staff must not be viewed as peripheral to the overall staffing of the executive office and the primary mission of the institution. Rather, fundraising, including the broader development goals of increasing visibility and friend-raising, need to be integrated into everything that occurs.

Adequate support for the fundraising activities of the institution is critical. The maxim it takes money to raise money is widely accepted. While the development budget will depend on the size of the institution and the resources available, it goes without saying that the development office must be financially accountable and fiscally prudent. There is no magic formula about how much money it takes to raise a million dollars; rather, the goal of the development staff and the executive should be to keep expenses for development within a very reasonable percentage of the money raised. It is generally recommended that development expenses should not exceed 15% of the goal of the fundraising effort. Thus, if the fundraising goal is $1 million, you should consider spending no more than $150,000 to reach that goal.

Up-front costs for development activities may be substantial, particularly if there is no previous history or organization of the volunteer activity. The initial investment in the start-up year may far exceed that which is obtained in gifts. But as previously mentioned, development is a long-term activity. Any investment in resources for fundraising for the present, assuming that the structures and processes are responsibly organized, will yield income in the future.

Establish organized systems for research and record-keeping and for financial accountability for the fundraising office. Research and record-keeping require sensitivity and, to the extent possible, the information obtained should be kept confidential, particularly as there often is information included about individuals that may be of a personal nature. All individuals who have access to any fundraising information should understand the confidential nature of the information. In cases where the donor has asked for anonymity in relation to their gift, the accounting system must be as confidential as possible. Professional development associations can provide guidelines to safeguard donor confidentiality and the inclusion of appropriate personal information in their donor files.

Success in fundraising requires adequate internal support for the professional fundraiser to engage primarily in solicitation activities. Other staff should be assigned the support activities, and there should be a clear acknowledgement that the fundraiser is to be held accountable for specific targets and goals.

WHEN SHOULD THE INSTITUTION SEEK A PROFESSIONAL CONSULTANT?

There are many fundraising consultants available to assist with the development activities, and as in most other areas, the fees vary with the level of expertise and the complexity of the project that the consultant is expected to undertake. It is important to have a formal contract with the consultant and to clearly understand the expectations, the deliverables, and the fee structure. While most consultants charge a basic fee, some consultants, in addition to the basic fee, charge a fee equal to some agreed-upon percentage of the funds raised. The executive must determine what level of consultation is needed, and at what price, in order to be successful in achieving the fundraising goals.

CHARACTERISTICS OF A DEVELOPMENT PROFESSIONAL

This profession is a little different from many others. Professional fundraisers should have a multitude of skills and talents. Some individuals think that professional fundraising is allied to sales, because it involves asking for the "order," and while there is not a quota or commission, there has to be an orientation to results. Marketing is a related profession, because there is an exchange between buyer and seller, and there needs to be some promotion or packaging of the program or project. Sometimes, the development professional provides financial information, as he/she presents options that have specific financial implications or tax savings benefits for the donor. All of these professionals have very distinctive characteristics and skill sets. The development professional needs to have some of the characteristics of each of these other professionals, as well as additional expertise.

First and foremost, there is the responsibility and privilege of representing a nonprofit organization. Development professionals must believe in the institution they represent. They must be knowledgeable about its programs or services, as well as the history of the organization. The professional must be credible and sincere. Along with a commitment to the institution, there must be a belief that there is a true benefit in supporting the institution they represent; that support will help this organization provide or meet a societal need, or promote better-quality life, for patients or individuals in the larger society.

While a type A personality is not a requirement or necessarily even preferred, a high energy level is needed. Usually there is some travel, even if local. Additionally, there are evening or early morning and weekend events that claim extra time and energy. The development professional needs to have a positive self-image. You are interacting with a wide range of individuals; occasionally, one will be rude or argumentative or, despite your very best efforts, refuse to become engaged. In this role, there needs to be an ongoing expectation of "Yes," but also the resilience to accept some rejection and not take it personally.

Management and organization skills are essential. The prospect pool must be constantly sorted, prioritized, and reprioritized. The coordination of prospect moves needs to be ongoing, determining who would be the most effective to see the prospect, the strategy, what activity should be planned, and under what timeline. Time management skills are a significant component. Along with deciding on which prospects to focus, it is often necessary to assign either self-imposed timelines, or those dictated by a campaign. There is always a need to move the prospect toward a gift.

As mentioned in previous chapters, listening skills are one of the most powerful tools any development professional can possess. Listening is a skill that takes practice, but can be honed. Along with the obvious benefits of clues for closing, it gives a valuable commodity—time—time to think, assimilate, and connect.

That brings us to another characteristic: the ability to think on one's feet and switch gears, sometimes in midstream. Hand and hand with this is creativity, not only to respond, but also to consider various options and perspectives and to make the best proposal or connection possible. The potential for synergy has become increasingly important to donors; they want to feel that they are getting the most bang for their buck.

It goes without saying that anyone who is involved in a development role should be interested in others; curious and caring about individuals' needs, wants, and desires. It is most helpful to seek to learn new ideas and perspectives in order to learn and grow in the understanding of your prospects.

For any development officer, what separates a good development professional from a truly excellent one is FOLLOW-THROUGH!! All of the most sophisticated systems for research and tracking, and sales skills, are ineffective if there is not timely follow-through.

The development professional should be comfortable with and able to accept a supporting role rather than the lead. There needs to be a willingness to put ego aside and allow others to have the spotlight. At times, the role can be analogous to that of producer or director.

Finally, a sense of humor enhances everything, and serves to ameliorate possible ulcers or anxiety attacks. The ability to laugh at yourself and see the humor in situations is a true gift, because to be effective, you need to enjoy what you are doing. Humor is a powerful medium.

The National Society of Fund Raising Executives (NSFRE) has developed standards describing the knowledge expected of senior fundraisers. In addition, many universities now offer courses and programs targeted to leadership in non-profit organizations; much of the content is centered on fundraising for the non-profits. It is expected that development professionals would have the knowledge in the following content areas: fundraising terminology; ethical aspects of fundraising; planned and deferred gifts; legal aspects of fundraising; interpersonal communication; and major gift solicitation techniques.

SUMMARY OF CHARACTERISTICS OF A DEVELOPMENT PROFESSIONAL

- Knowledge of fundraising basics;
- Skill and experience in gift solicitation;
- Excellent interpersonal skills;
- Excellent organizational skills;
- High energy level;
- Keen interest in others;
- Curiosity;
- Flexibility;
- Comfort with a supporting role;
- Sense of humor; and
- Commitment and loyalty.

SUMMARY OF REQUIREMENTS FOR A SUCCESSFUL AND EFFICIENT DEVELOPMENT OFFICE

- Adequate financial resources;
- Professional fundraising staff;
- Adequate support staff;
- Access to planned giving and legal expertise; and
- Systems for research and tracking of the development efforts.

DEVELOPMENT OFFICER'S PERSPECTIVE

It is incumbent on the development officer to assess the fundraising needs of the organization and to make realistic recommendations for staff, direct costs, and indirect costs, such as travel, equipment, and supplies. On this basis, there is a context for revenue projections. A start-up situation, naturally, will require more up-front costs, as will a campaign. For new or expanding operations, there might be a phase-in projection or plan.

The most important consideration is setting realistic expectations of outcomes. If it is a one-person office, this needs to be considered in delegating assignments, and be reflected in fundraising goals. Establish the percentage of time the development officer is to devote to direct fundraising and how much to other responsibilities. In a school setting, there is a tendency for some deans to involve the development officer in a number of other events or activities outside of the development initiative. This is the prerogative of the dean but with each assignment of such activities, it dilutes the focus on development. Remember, calls equal cash.

To maximize the effectiveness of the development officer, some staff support is needed. Perhaps an executive's assistant could be asked to devote a portion of his/her time to the operation. If resources are limited, a volunteer could be recruited to coordinate the annual fund drive, working with the development officer and dean. This would enable the dean and development officer to concentrate on major gift activity and targeted foundation and corporate proposals. In one of my past positions, I had the great good fortune to have a member of the Board of Trustees volunteer clerical and administrative support a couple of days each week.

Development is an investment of time and resources, not a quick fix. Developing an effective and efficient fundraising operation is a valuable asset for an organization and is fast becoming a necessity.

DEAN OR EXECUTIVE'S PERSPECTIVE

Next to your secretary or administrative assistant, the development officer will know you best. He/she should have total access to your calendar, and you should feel free to discuss the details of the work situation and the goals of the institution with the development officer. Development officers can help you frame the fundraising in relation to the strengths of the institution as well and build on your strengths in the cycle of solicitation, cultivation, and stewardship of donors.

Appendices

A. Sample Gift Table

B. Resources and Bibliography for Fundraising

C. Endowed Chairs Articles
   1. Fitzpatrick, J. J. (2000). Endowed chairs and professorships in schools of nursing: A 1999 update. *Journal of Professional Nursing, 16,* 57–62.
   2. Fitzpatrick, J. J., & Carnegie, M. E. (1991). Endowed chairs in nursing. *Nursing Outlook, 39,* 218–221.

D. Fundraising Articles
   1. Deller, S. S., & Fitzpatrick, J. J. (1997). Primer for philanthropy: The ABCs of fundraising. *Nursing Leadership Forum, 3,* 98–101.
   2. Fitzpatrick, J. J. (1996). Twelve principles of successful fund-raising. *Nursing Leadership Forum, 1,* 4–7.

E. Fundraising Reports from the Council for Aid to Education (Web site: www.cae.org)

Appendix A

Sample Gift Table

Sample Gift Table: Assumes Development Goal of $25,000,000

Type	Gift level	Number of donors	Total
Major gifts	$2,500,000	1	$2,500,000
	1,000,000	4	4,000,000
	500,000	4	2,000,000
	250,000	6	1,500,000
	150,000	10	1,500,000
	100,000	23	2,300,000
Special gifts	50,000	42	2,100,000
	25,000	54	1,350,000
	10,000	135	1,350,000
General campaign	5,000	420	2,100,000
	1,000	2,100	2,100,000
	under 1,000	33,000	2,200,000
Total		35,799	$25,000,000

Appendix B

Resources and Bibliography for Fundraising

INSTITUTIONS AND ASSOCIATIONS

Council for Advancement in Support of Education (CASE)
1307 New York Avenue NW, Suite 1000
Washington, DC 20005
(202) 328-5900
Fax: (202) 387-4973
http://www.case.org

Includes 3000 institutional members; approximately 15,000 development professionals receive benefits through these institutional members. A directory of members is available. CASE also publishes guidelines for gift accounting.

National Society of Fund Raising Executives (NSFRE)
1101 King Street, Suite 700
Alexandria VA 22314
(703) 684-0410 or 1-800 688-FIND
Fax: (703) 684-0540

Provides information about fundraising to members; includes a library with resources catalogues according to interest area, such as giving among women or among the elderly.

Council for Aid to Education (CAE)
342 Madison Avenue, Suite 1532
New York, NY 10173
(212) 661-5800
Fax: (212) 661-9766
http://www.cae.org

An independent subsidiary of RAND; publishes an annual report of Voluntary Support of Education; prepares several tables and charts detailing giving trends.

Council on Foundations
1828 L Street NW
Washington, DC 20036
(202) 466-6512
Fax: (202) 785-3926
www.cof.org

A not-for-profit membership organization which provides information on grant making among foundations and corporations.

Foundation Center (5 physical sites available)
79 Fifth Avenue
New York, NY 10003
(212) 620-4230
Fax: (212) 691-1828

1001 Connecticut Avenue, NW, Suite 938
Washington, DC 20036
(202) 331-1400
Fax: (202) 331-1739

1422 Euclid, Suite 1356
Cleveland, OH 44155
(216) 861-1933
Fax: 861-1936

312 Sutter Street, Room 312
San Francisco, CA 94108
(415) 397-0902
Fax: (415) 397-7670

Hurt Building, 50 Hurt Plaza
Grand Lobby, Suite 150
Atlanta, GA 30303
(404) 880-0094
Fax: (404) 880-0097
www.fdncenter.org

The Foundation Center has a library available and staff to assist with questions in each of its five locations. Included in the resources available from The Foundation Center are *The Foundation Directory, The Foundation Grants Index, The Guide to U.S. Foundations, The National Directory of Corporate Giving*, and *A User-Friendly Guide: A Grantseeker's Guide to Resources*

Philanthropy: A publication of The Philanthropy Roundtable
1150 17th Street, NW
Washington, DC 20036
(202) 822-8333
Fax: (202) 822-8325
www.philanthrophyroundtable.org

Serves as a resource of news and information for grantmakers, and a forum for donors to communicate with one another about programs, ideas, and experiences in philanthropy.

The Philanthropy Roundtable is a national association of individual donors, corporate giving representatives, foundation staff and trustees, and trust and estate officers. The Roundtable also sponsors regional meetings, holds an annual national conference, and offers referral services for donors who seek advice on managing giving programs and starting and maintaining foundations.

The Chronicle of Philanthropy: The Newspaper of the Nonprofit World
1255 23rd Street, NW
Washington, DC 20037
(202) 466-1200
www.philanthropy.com

Serves as a key source of information about issues relevant to philanthropy, including timely reports on top funders and sources of support. Through the *Chronicle* Web site, one can register for a subscription to a funding source which can search foundations and corporations, using keywords, to determine what has been funded in a particular area. Also available is information on seminars and workshops, conferences, etc.

National Committee on Planned Giving
233 McCrea Street, Suite 400
Indianapolis, IN 46225
(317) 269-6274
Fax: (317) 269-6276
www.ncpg.org

Publishes *Gift Planner Update*, a newsletter distributed to more than 10,000 gift planners, which includes helpful tips for fundraising through gift planning.

University Programs
Indiana University Center on Philanthropy
550 West North Street, Suite 301
Indianapolis, IN 46202-3162
(317) 684-8922
Fax: (317) 684-8900
www.tcop.org

Provides a broad spectrum of knowledge and critical thought on the topic of philanthropy through book and essay publication and seminars and courses.

INTERNET RESOURCES

Web sites that review or rank reputable charities:

GuideStar (www.guidestar.com) includes 620,000 nonprofit organizations in its database, and is the Web's most comprehensive list of charities. It does not include an evaluation of the charities for either quality or reputation.

National Charities Information Bureau (www.give.org) rates 400 charities based on the NCIB's own financial reporting criteria.

American Institute of Philanthropy (www.charitywatch.org) covers a few hundred charities, noting the ones that have opened their books to the organization, and those that put more than 75% of their revenues toward programs rather than administrative support.

Philanthropic Advisory Service of the Better Business Bureau (www.bbb. org/about.pas.html) offers profiles on a few hundred charities, noting their compliance status with the BBB's standards.

SOFTWARE RESOURCES

Connections, a new computer database application, was designed to track "who knows whom" and to show what organizations each of those people influence. *Connections* tracks other details that are associated with development contacts. For example, *Connections* stores an individual contact's banking service providers, interests, organizations influenced, and positions held on influential committees. Also, *Connections* tracks many factors related to the organizations that a development contact is associated with such as: the organization's budget, mission, programs, banking service providers, and more. Among other printed reports, *Connections* shows at a glance which person knows which people and what organizations those people influence. A data-driven graphic is provided by *Connections* that portrays the range of influence of development contacts contained in the database. A graph ranks individuals with most influence based on number of contacts with other influential people. This program can increase productivity and enhance the organization of data related to friend-raising and fundraising. A label subsystem is also provided, which facilitates mail lists for events, activities, and communication updates.

   Connections is a computer program that runs under Microsoft Access 97 or Microsoft Access 2000 on a Local Area Network or on a stand-alone PC.
For more information, please contact:
John M. Walker
Hinton Walker Associates at 303.713.9175
email may be sent to johnwalker50@msn.com
Postal mail may be sent to:
Hinton Walker Associates
5367 E. Mineral Circle
Littleton, CO 80122
Fax: 303.713.9177

CASE INTRODUCTORY BIBLIOGRAPHY
FUNDRAISING

Here is a sampling of the materials available from CASE and other sources. CURRENTS and other CASE publications are available on numerous topics in addition to those cited here. Back issues of CASE CURRENTS and copies of other case publications may be purchased by calling the CASE Publications Order Department (800) 554-8536 or (301) 604-2068, or FAX (301) 206-9789.

- Brittingham, Barbara E. and Thomas R. Pezzullo. *The Campus Green: Fund Raising in Higher Education.* ASHE-ERIC Higher Education Report, 1990. [Cooperative project of the Council for Advancement and Support of Education and the ERIC Clearinghouse on Higher Education, and available for purchase from CASE].
- Buchanan, Peter McE. "Some Blunt Talk about Fund Raising: Council for Advancement and Support of Education's President Talks about Why Advancement Officers Need to Rethink, Restructure, and Communicate Anew about Their Fund-Raising Campaigns," *CURRENTS* (October 1991): 10.
- Costello, Kathryn R. "What I Expect From My CEO: A Chief Advancement Officer Outlines the Qualities That Make a President or Head an Ally in Fund Raising," *CURRENTS* (November/December 1993): 24.
- Council for Advancement and Support of Education. *Donor Bill of Rights.* Washington, DC: Council for Advancement and Support of Education and others, 1994.
- Council for Advancement and Support of Education. *Case Management Reporting Standards: Standards for Annual Giving and Campaigns in Educational Fund Raising.* Washington, DC: Council for Advancement and Support of Education, 1996.
- Council for Aid to Education. *Voluntary Support of Education: National Trends.* [Annual survey] New York, NY: Council for Aid to Education. [Cosponsored by CASE and NAIS].
- Dunlop, David and Ellen Ryan. "Thirty Years in Fund Raising: Master Fund Raiser David Dunlop Tells What He's Learned about the Staff's Role in Dealing with Donors," *CURRENTS* (November/December 1990): 32.

- Faust, Paula. *An Introduction to Fund Raising: A Newcomer's Guide to Development.* Washington, DC: Council for Advancement and Support of Education, 1983.
- Fisher, James and Gary H. Quehl. *The President and Fund Raising.* Phoenix, AZ: ACE/Oryx Press, 1989. [Available for purchase from Council for Advancement and Support of Education].
- Gee, Ann D. *Annual Giving Strategies: A Comprehensive Guide to Better Results.* Washington, DC: Council for Advancement and Support of Education, 1990.
- Hodgkinson, Virginia and others. *Giving and Volunteering in the United States: Findings from a National Survey.* Washington, DC: Independent Sector, 1994.
- Jones, Jeremy. *A Development Handbook: Promoting Philanthropy at Independent Schools.* Washington, DC: Council for Advancement and Support of Education, 1992.
- Kelly, Kathleen S. *Fund Raising and Public Relations: A Critical Analysis.* Lawrence Erlbaum Associates, 1991. [Available for purchase from Council for Advancement and Support of Education].
- Lowery, William R. "Divide and Conquer: Pairing the Right Trustee with the Right Task Will Make Board Members a More Effective Part of Your Development Team," *CURRENTS* (September 1993): 41.
- Matheny, Richard E. *Major Gifts: Solicitation Strategies.* Washington, DC: Council for Advancement and Support of Education, 1994.
- Pezzullo, Thomas and Barbara E. Brittingham. "The Study of Money: What We Know and What We Need to Know about College Fund Raising," *CURRENTS* (July/August 1990): 44.
- Quigg, H. Gerald. *The Successful Capital Campaign: From Planning to Victory Celebration.* Washington, DC: Council for Advancement and Support of Education, 1986.
- Ryan, Ellen. "Annual Fund Answers: Experts in Direct Mail. Phonathons, and In-Person Asks Tackle Some of the Annual Fund's Perennial Problems," *CURRENTS* (May 1996): 30.
- Ryan, Ellen. "The Cost of Raising a Dollar: A Four-Year Study Has Produced Workable Standards for Capturing Comparative Costs Useful to Leaders in Fund Raising. Alumni Administration, and Public Relations," *CURRENTS* (September 1990): 58.
- Ryan, Ellen. "Sticky Wickets: Fund Raisers Face Questions of Right or Wrong Every Day. Here's How Council for Advancement and Support of Education Professionals Would Handle Six Ethical Conundrums in Development," *CURRENTS* (July/August 1993): 58.

- Ryan, G. Jeremiah and Nanette J. Smith. *Marketing and Development for Community Colleges.* Washington, DC: Council for Advancement and Support of Education, 1989.
- Seymour, Harold J. *Designs for Fund Raising: Principles, Patterns, and Techniques.* Rockville, MD: Taft Group, 1988. [Available for purchase from Council for Advancement and Support of Education].
- Shoemaker, Donna. *Greenbriar II: A Look at the Future: A Report on the Council for Advancement and Support of Education Colloquium on Professionalism in Institutional Advancement.* The Greenbriar, February 13–15, 1985. Washington, DC: Council for Advancement and Support of Education, 1985.
- Terrell, Melvin and James A. Gold. *New Roles for Educational Fundraising and Institutional Advancement.* New Directions for Student Services Series, no. 63. San Francisco, CA: Jossey-Bass Publishers, Fall 1993.
- U.S. Department of Education. *Digest of Education Statistics, 1995.* Washington, DC: U.S. Department of Education, Office of Educational Research and Improvement, National Center for Education Statistics, 1995.
- Unkefer, Jane and Paul Chewning. *Institutional Advancement Professional Area Guide.* Washington, DC: Council for Advancement and Support of Education, 1992.
- Williams, Roger L. "Advancement's Steady Advance: Demographics Stay the Course, Salaries Rise, But Pay Gaps Persist, According to the Fourth CASE Survey of Institutional Advancement" *CURRENTS* (February 1996): 8.
- Worth, Michael J. *Educational Fund Raising: Principles and Practice.* Phoenix, AZ: ACE/Oryx Press, 1993. [Available for purchase from Case].

Appendix C

Endowed Chairs Articles

Endowed Chairs and Professorships in Schools of Nursing: A 1999 Update

JOYCE J. FITZPATRICK, PHD, RN, FAAN*

SINCE 1984, when the first survey of endowed chairs in schools of nursing was published (Fitzpatrick, 1985), the number of recorded chairs has increased from 20 as of 1984 to 167 as of the first half of 1999. The 1990s have been particularly productive: many schools have enhanced their development efforts and thus substantially increased their private funding, including funding for endowed chairs. The increase in the numbers of chairs since the 1995 publication of the survey results (Fitzpatrick, 1995) is in itself impressive. From 1995 through the first half of 1999, 64 new chairs and professorships have been funded in schools of nursing.

Several aspects of the survey data are noteworthy. First, deans were contacted to determine the initial endowment amount that was committed at the date that the professorship/chair was officially named. To the extent that the author has been able to determine, this is the amount reported in column three of Table 1. It is prominent that, even with endowments committed in the same year, there are major differences in the total amounts. This variation can be attributed to differences in the college and university requirements for named professorships or chairs. In some universities, a smaller amount is required for an endowed professorship compared with an endowed chair. In other universities, there is no distinction made between endowed professorships and endowed chairs. Also, it can be noted from the data reported in Table 1 that there generally is an increase in the amount of an endowed professorship/chair as the years progress. For example, the amount required for an endowed chair in many of the top universities at this time is

$1.5 million. Ten years ago, $1 million might have sufficed.

Although the focus of this survey was to determine the initial amount required to fund a professorship/chair, in the process of collecting the data two other aspects of the increase in endowment funding to schools of nursing were noted. First, the current market value of the endowments for some of these professorships/chairs is much larger than the original endowment. Both Vanderbilt and Johns Hopkins Schools of Nursing, for example, report market values of some of their chairs as $2 to $3 million. Two factors can contribute to such substantial increases in market value: good returns on investments and reinvestments of all of the accumulated interest as a result of not filling the position. In the next survey, an effort will be made to report current market value in addition to the original amount of the endowment. Second, several schools reported future commitments of endowed chairs; these will be reported in future articles.

Another aspect of the most recently funded professorships/chairs is notable. Many schools have named chairs after contemporary nurse leaders, particularly those who played a significant role in leadership for that particular school. Examples include the chairs named after Claire Fagin at Penn, Bernardine Lacey at Western Michigan, Rhetaugh Dumas at University of Michigan, Erline McGriff at New York University, Loretta Ford at University of Colorado, Mary Harper at Tuskegee University, Jeannette Lancaster at the University of Virginia, and Harriet Werley at the University of Illinois.

In summary, schools of nursing have made much progress in the last 25 years in garnering outside private resources to support the academic mission. Furthermore, it is expected that as the level of awareness of nursing education and professional practice increases through advancements in public support for nursing, there will be a concomitant increase in private funding.

*Professor, School of Nursing, Case Western Reserve University, Cleveland, OH; and Visiting Scholar, New York University and Mount Sinai Hospital, New York, NY.

From *Journal of Professional Nursing*, Vol 16, No 1 (January–February), 2000: pp 57–62. Reprinted by permission of W. B. Saunders, a Harcourt Health Sciences Company.

TABLE 1. Summary of Endowed Chairs and Professorships in Schools of Nursing

School	Date of Initial Endowment	Amount of Initial Endowment ($)	Focus	Name
University of Virginia School of Nursing	1926	50,000	Nursing education	Sadie Heath Cabaniss
University of Cincinnati College of Nursing and Health	1948	217,000	Graduate education	Jane E. Procter
Illinois Wesleyan University School of Nursing	1961	*	Not specified	Caroline F. Rupert
University of South Carolina Columbia College of Nursing	1965	144,000	Community health	Emily Myrtle Smith
University of Washington School of Nursing	1965	250,000	Health promotion	Elizabeth Sterling Soule
University of Cincinnati College of Nursing and Health	1968	250,000	Dean	Jacob J. Schmidlapp
University of Wisconsin-Madison School of Nursing	1971	1,000,000	Research and teaching	Helen Denne Schulte
University of Wisconsin-Madison School of Nursing	1971	1,000,000	Research and teaching	Helen Denne Schulte
Hartwick College Department of Nursing	1973	500,000	Nursing	A. Lindsay and Olive B. O'Connor
Vanderbilt University School of Nursing	1975	1,175,000	Not specified	Valere Potter
North Park College Division of Nursing	1977	500,000	Nursing	Paul W. Brandel
University of Iowa College of Nursing	1977	1,200,000	Nursing	Kelting
Columbia University Teachers College	1979	230,000	Nursing education	Isabel Maitland Stewart
Rush University College of Nursing	1979	2,000,000	Dean	John L. and Helen Kellogg
University of North Carolina—Chapel Hill School of Nursing	1979	200,000	Thanatology	Carol Ann Beerstecher Blackwell
Loyola University Marcella Neihoff School of Nursing	1980	500,000	Nursing research	Neihoff
Ashland University School of Nursing	1981	500,000	Dean	Hugo and Mabel B. Young
Case Western Reserve University Frances Payne Bolton School of Nursing	1981	750,000	Gerontological nursing	Florence Cellar
University of Pennsylvania School of Nursing	1981	600,000	Psychiatric nursing	van Ameringen
Avila College Department of Nursing	1982	250,000	Chairperson of nursing	Hallmark
Incarnate Word College Division of Nursing	1982	400,000	Research	Lillian Dunlap
Louisiana College Department of Nursing	1982	500,000	Nursing	Coughlin-Saunders
University of Minnesota School of Nursing	1982	1,000,000	Nursing research	Cora Meidl Siehl
University of Nevada-Reno Orvis School of Nursing	1982	750,000	Graduate education	Arthur Emerton Orvis
University of Texas at Austin School of Nursing	1982	100,000	Faculty recognition	La Quinta Motor Inns, Inc
University of Texas at Austin School of Nursing	1982	100,000	Faculty recognition	Luci B. Johnson
University of Texas at Austin School of Nursing	1982	100,000	Faculty recognition	James R. Dougherty, Jr
Case Western Reserve University Frances Payne Bolton School of Nursing	1983	750,000	Community health nursing	Kate Hanna Harvey
University of Miami School of Nursing	1983	1,000,000	Transcultural nursing	William R. Ryan
University of Texas at Austin School of Nursing	1983	100,000	Faculty recognition	Joseph H. Blades
University of Texas at Austin School of Nursing	1983	100,000	Faculty recognition	Denton and Louise Cooley
Case Western Reserve University Frances Payne Bolton School of Nursing	1984	2,100,000	Nursing	Edward and Louise Mellen
Frontier Nursing Service School of Nurse-Midwifery and Family Nursing	1984	595,000	Nurse-midwifery	Mary Breckinridge
The Johns Hopkins University School of Nursing	1984	1,400,000	Clinical nursing	M. Adelaide Nutting
Oregon Health Sciences School of Nursing	1984	2,021,000	Nursing research	Nursing research

(Continued on following page)

TABLE 1. Summary of Endowed Chairs and Professorships in Schools of Nursing (Cont'd)

School	Date of Initial Endowment	Amount of Initial Endowment ($)	Focus	Name
University of Maryland School of Nursing	1984	1,500,000	Gerontological nursing	Sonya Ziporkin Gershowitz
University of Wisconsin-Madison School of Nursing	1984	550,000	Not specified	Bascom-Moehlman
Adelphi University School of Nursing	1985	500,000	Not specified	Vera E. Bender
Florida Atlantic University College of Nursing	1985	1,000,000	Not specified	Christine E. Lynn
University of Florida-Gainesville College of Nursing	1985	1,262,000	Oncology nursing	Kirbo
University of Oklahoma College of Nursing	1985	1,377,000	Gerontological nursing	Parry
University of Wisconsin-Milwaukee School of Nursing	1985	1,000,000	Nursing research	Walter Schroeder
Texas Woman's University College of Nursing	1986	500,000	Health promotion and disease prevention	Parry
University of California-San Francisco School of Nursing	1986	700,000	Research with direct impact on patient care	James P. and Marjorie A. Livingston
University of South Florida College of Nursing	1986	1,000,000	Nursing education and scholarship	Southwest Florida
Florida Gulf Coast University Department of Nursing	1987	2,900,000	Innovative and futuristic nursing programs	Southwest Florida
The Johns Hopkins University School of Nursing	1987	1,000,000	Clinical nursing	Elsie M. Lawler
Case Western Reserve University Frances Payne Bolton School of Nursing	1988	1,000,000	Nursing	Elizabeth Brooks Ford
Massachusetts General Hospital Institute of Health Professions	1988	1,000,000	Nursing research	Amelia Peabody
Tuskegee University School of Nursing	1988	500,000	Mental health/aging	Mary Starke Harper
University of Memphis Loewenberg School of Nursing	1988	1,000,000	Excellence in nursing	William A. and Ruth F. Loewenberg
University of Missouri-Columbia School of Nursing	1988	351,500	Excellence in nursing	Potter-Brinton
University of Pennsylvania School of Nursing	1988	1,500,000	Leadership	Margaret Bond Simon
University of Texas at Austin School of Nursing	1988	500,000	Dean	Laura Lee Blanton
University of Texas Health Sciences Center at Houston School of Nursing	1988	500,000	Gerontological nursing	Isla Carroll Turner
Case Western Reserve University Frances Payne Bolton School of Nursing	1989	1,000,000	Nursing education	Independence Foundation
Emory University Nell Hodgson School of Nursing	1989	1,000,000	Nursing education	Independence Foundation
The Johns Hopkins University School of Nursing	1989	1,000,000	Nursing education	Independence Foundation
New York University Division of Nursing	1989	1,000,000	Nursing education	Independence Foundation
Rush University College of Nursing	1989	1,000,000	Nursing education	Independence Foundation
University of Minnesota School of Nursing	1989	500,000	Long-term care	Long-term care
University of Pennsylvania School of Nursing	1989	1,000,000	Nursing education	Independence Foundation
University of Rochester School of Nursing	1989	1,000,000	Nursing education	Independence Foundation
University of South Carolina-Spartanburg Mary Black School of Nursing	1989	100,000	Caregiving in AIDS research	Jimmy A. Ferrell, PhD
University of Virginia School of Nursing	1989	100,000	Chronic illness	Madge M. Jones
Vanderbilt University School of Nursing	1989	1,000,000	Nursing education	Independence Foundation
Virginia Commonwealth University School of Nursing	1989	750,000	Nursing	Centennial
Yale University School of Nursing	1989	1,000,000	Nursing education	Independence Foundation

(Continued on following page)

TABLE 1. Summary of Endowed Chairs and Professorships in Schools of Nursing (Cont'd)

School	Date of Initial Endowment	Amount of Initial Endowment ($)	Focus	Name
Columbia College Department of Nursing	1990	95,000	Not specified	Marjorie Wolff German
Columbia University School of Nursing	1990	1,500,000	Health policy	Centennial
Emory University Nell Hodgson Woodruff School of Nursing	1990	1,000,000	Oncology	Edith Folsom Honeycutt
Northeast Louisiana University School of Nursing	1990	100,000	Teaching and research	Glenwood Regional Medical Center
University of Central Florida College of Health and Public Affairs	1990	1,000,000	Nursing education	Bert Fish
University of Pennsylvania School of Nursing	1990	1,250,000	Leadership	Claire M. Fagin
University of South Carolina-Columbia College of Nursing	1990	110,000	Oncology nursing	Dunn-Shealy
University of Utah College of Nursing	1990	1,250,000	Research	Louis S. Peery, M.D., and Janet B. Peery
Vanderbilt University School of Nursing	1990	508,000	Not specified	Julia Eleanor Blair Chenault
Yale University School of Nursing	1990	1,000,000	Nursing	Annie W. Goodrich
University of North Carolina-Chapel Hill School of Nursing	1991	650,000	Nursing research	Francis Hill Fox
University of Pennsylvania School of Nursing	1991	300,000	Not specified	Helen Shearer
Case Western Reserve University Frances Payne Bolton School of Nursing	1992	1,200,000	Pediatric nursing	Carl W. and Margaret Davis Walter
Columbia University School of Nursing	1992	1,500,000	Nursing research	Anna C. Maxwell
Columbia University School of Nursing	1992	1,700,000	Not specified	Alumni
Saint Louis University School of Nursing	1992	1,000,000	Nursing research	
University of Alabama Birmingham School of Nursing	1992	1,400,000	Nursing research	Marie L. O'Koren
University of North Carolina-Charlotte College of Nursing and Health Professions	1992	500,000	Research	Dean W. Colvard
University of Wisconsin-Madison School of Nursing	1992	1,000,000	Not specified	Charlotte J. and Ralph A. Rodefer
Austin Peay State University School of Nursing	1993	1,250,000	Excellence in nursing	Lenona C. Reuther
The Johns Hopkins University School of Nursing	1993	1,000,000	Not specified	Anna D. Wolf
Northeast Louisiana University School of Nursing	1993	100,000	Research	Lawton
Northeast Louisiana University School of Nursing	1993	100,000	Teaching and research	NLU Foundation
Prairie View A & M College of Nursing	1993	1,500,000	Minority health and research	Houston Endowment, Inc
University of Hawaii at Manoa School of Nursing	1993	1,500,000	Woman's health	Frances A. Matsuda
University of Virginia School of Nursing	1993	250,000	Clinical research	Betty Norman Norris
Binghamton University Decker School of Nursing	1994	1,000,000	Community health nursing	Decker
Case Western Reserve University Frances Payne Bolton School of Nursing	1994	750,000	Oncology nursing	Gertrude Perkins Oliva
Columbia University School of Nursing	1994	1,500,000	Pharmaceutical and therapeutic research	Pharmaceutical and Therapeutic Research
Columbia University School of Nursing	1994	1,500,000	International nursing	Henrik H. Bendixen
Northeast Louisiana University School of Nursing	1994	100,000	Teaching and research	Twohig
University of California-Los Angeles School of Nursing	1994	350,000	Nursing research	Lulu Wolf Hassenplug
University of Michigan School of Nursing	1994	1,200,000	Nursing systems research	Rhetaugh Graves Dumas
University of Missouri-St. Louis Barnes College of Nursing	1994	1,100,000	Nursing	Hubert C. Moog

(Continued on following page)

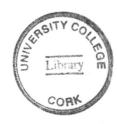

TABLE 1. Summary of Endowed Chairs and Professorships in Schools of Nursing (Cont'd)

School	Date of Initial Endowment	Amount of Initial Endowment ($)	Focus	Name
University of Pennsylvania School of Nursing	1994	1,000,000	Community care	Viola McInnes
University of Texas-Houston School of Nursing	1994	100,000	Aging	Theodore J. and Mary E. Trumble
University of Washington School of Nursing	1994	100,000	Faculty recognition	Charles and Gerda Spence
Columbia University School of Nursing	1995	750,000	Not specified	Elizabeth Standish Gill
University of Nebraska College of Nursing	1995	1,000,000	Community family and/or women's health	Dorothy Hodges Olsen
University of Pennsylvania School of Nursing	1995	1,250,000	Gerontological nursing	Edith Clemmer Steinbright
University of Pennsylvania School of Nursing	1995	1,250,000	Medical-surgical nursing	Lillian S. Bruner
University of Pennsylvania School of Nursing	1995	1,250,000	Nursing	
University of Pennsylvania School of Nursing	1995	250,000		Ralston House
University of South Florida School of Nursing	1995	1,000,000	Nursing informatics	Lewis and Leona Hughes
University of Virginia School of Nursing	1995	400,000	Primary care	Theresa A. Thomas
Capstone College of Nursing	1996	*	Rural nursing	Martha Lucinda Luher
Case Western Reserve University Frances Payne Bolton School of Nursing	1996	2,300,000	Care of vulnerable and at-risk persons	John Burry, Jr
Columbia University School of Nursing	1996	750,000	Not specified	Helen F. Pettit
Columbia University School of Nursing	1996	1,000,000	Oncology	
New Jersey University of Medicine and Dentistry Department of Nursing	1996	1,300,000	Community pediatric nursing	Francois-Xavier Bagnoud
University of Illinois-Chicago College of Nursing	1996	1,500,000	Nursing research	harriet H. Werley
University of Texas-Houston School of Nursing	1996	250,000	Oncology nursing	John S. Dunn, Sr
University of Texas-Houston School of Nursing	1996	250,000	Nursing	John P. McGovern
University of Washington School of Nursing	1996	250,000	Aging	Aljoya
Emory University School of Nursing	1997	250,000	Not specified	Betty Tigner Turner
Pennsylvania State University School of Nursing	1997	500,000	Community service	Elouise Ross Eberly
Pennsylvania State University School of Nursing	1997	500,000	Research	Elouise Ross Eberly
University of Alabama-Birmingham School of Nursing	1997	1,100,000	Aging	
University of Nebraska College of Nursing	1997	1,000,000	Not specified	Charlotte Peck Lienemann and alumni
University of Pennsylvania School of Nursing	1997	350,000	Not specified	Miriam Stirl
University of Texas-El Paso School of Nursing	1997	1,600,000	Community health	Charles and Shirley Leavell
University of Texas-Houston School of Nursing	1997	250,000	Nursing	Lee and Joseph Jamail
University of Texas-Houston School of Nursing	1997	250,000	Nursing	Lee and Joseph Jamail
University of Texas-Houston School of Nursing	1997	250,000	Nursing	Lee and Joseph Jamail
University of Utah College of Nursing	1997	1,250,000	Women's and reproductive health	Annette Poulson Cumming
Boston College School of Nursing	1998	1,000,000	Nursing scholarship	Lelia Holden Carroll
Indiana University School of Nursing	1998	500,000	Pediatric oncology	Holmquist
Medical College of Georgia School of Nursing	1998	860,000	Nursing	Kellett
University of Arizona College of Nursing	1998	500,000	Not specified	Gladys E. Sorensen

(Continued on following page)

TABLE 1. Summary of Endowed Chairs and Professorships in Schools of Nursing (Cont'd)

School	Date of Initial Endowment	Amount of Initial Endowment ($)	Focus	Name
University of California-Los Angeles School of Nursing	1998	500,000	Nursing science	Adrienne Moseley
University of California-San Francisco School of Nursing	1998	700,000	Nursing education	
University of California-San Francisco School of Nursing	1998	500,000	Nursing education	Nursing alumni and Mary Harm
University of Colorado School of Nursing	1998	1,500,000	Caring science	Murchison-Scorville
University of Colorado School of Nursing	1998	1,500,000	Pediatric nursing	The Children's Hospital
University of Colorado School of Nursing	1998	1,500,000	Nurse practitioner	Loretta C. Ford
University of Michigan School of Nursing	1998	1,200,000	Oncology nursing	Mary Lou Willard French
University of South Florida School of Nursing	1998	100,000	Acute care	Gordon Keller
University of Missouri-Columbia Sinclair School of Nursing	1998	1,100,000	Gerontological nursing and public policy	Millsap
University of Texas-Austin School of Nursing	1998	100,000	Faculty recognition	Jamil
University of Texas Health Science Center at San Antonio School of Nursing	1998	1,200,000	Research	Nursing Research
University of Texas-Houston School of Nursing	1998	100,000	Addictions nursing	John P. McGovern
University of Utah College of Nursing	1998	1,250,000	Gerontological nursing	Helen Lowe Bamberger Colby
University of Washington School of Nursing	1998	250,000	Health promotion	Elizabeth Sterling Soule
Western Michigan School of Nursing	1998	1,500,000	Community health nursing	Bernardine Lacey
Case Western Reserve University Frances Payne Bolton School of Nursing	1999	1,250,000	Not specified	Sarah Cole Hirsh
New York University Division of Nursing	1999	1,500,000	Division head	Erline Perkins McGriff
Oakland University School of Nursing	1999	1,000,000	Geriatrics and rehabilitation	Maggie Allesee
University of Florida College of Nursing	1999	1,000,000	Nursing excellence	A. Jenks
University of Kentucky School of Nursing	1999	1,000,000	Cardiovascular and/or pulmonary health care	Linda C. Gill
University of Kentucky School of Nursing	1999	750,000	Community health	Good Samaritan
University of Kentucky School of Nursing	1999	200,000	Individuals, families, and/or communities at risk	Marcia A. Dake
University of Kentucky School of Nursing	1999	100,000	Leadership	Commonwealth
University of Pittsburgh School of Nursing	1999	1,500,000	Nursing science	UPMC Health System
University of South Florida School of Nursing	1999	100,000	Oncology nursing	Beatrice Thompson
University of Utah College of Nursing	1999	1,250,000	Not specified	Ida May "Dotty" Barnes, RN, and D. Keith Barnes, MD
University of Utah College of Nursing	1999	1,250,000	Not specified	Louis H. Peery
University of Virginia School of Nursing	1999	500,000	Nursing	UVA Medical Center
University of Virginia School of Nursing	1999	500,000	Nursing	Jeannette Lancaster and alumni
Wayne State University College of Nursing	1999	800,000	Not specified	Katherine Faville

NOTE: Data are presented in chronological order according to year of endowment.

Abbreviations: AIDS, acquired immunodeficiency virus syndrome; NLU, Northeast Louisiana University; UPMC, University of Pittsburgh Medical Center; UVA, University of Virginia.

*Amount not determined.

References

Fitzpatrick, J. J. (1985). Endowed chairs in nursing: State of the art. *Journal of Professional Nursing, 1,* 145-147.

Fitzpatrick, J. J. (1989). Endowed chairs in nursing: A 1988 update. *Journal of Professional Nursing, 5,* 23-24.

Fitzpatrick, J. J. (1995). We've come a long way: A 1995 report of endowed chairs in nursing. *Journal of Professional Nursing, 11,* 320-324.

ENDOWED CHAIRS IN NURSING

Two distinguished scholars discuss aspects of endowed chairs: Joyce Fitzpatrick provides a brief history of the practice and explains how endowed chairs preserve academic freedom and nursing's place in scientific inquiry. M. Elizabeth Carnegie recounts a brief history of endowed chairs in the U.S. and relates her own experiences gained from filling endowed chairs in nursing.

by Joyce J. Fitzpatrick and M. Elizabeth Carnegie

ENDOWED CHAIRS: OPPORTUNITY FOR ACADEMIC FREEDOM
Joyce J. Fitzpatrick

Nursing is an art; and if it is to be made an art, it requires as exclusive a devotion, as hard a preparation, as any painter's or sculptor's work; for what is the having to do with dead canvas or cold marble, compared with having to do with the living body...it is one of the Fine Arts; I had almost said, the finest of the Fine Arts.—Florence Nightingale

Perhaps, if Florence were alive today, she would indeed conclude, as we have, that not only is nursing the finest art, but so also is it an important scientific scholarly enterprise. Our focus on endowed chairs in nursing is a symbol of our advancements within the great universities in our nation, for an endowed chair is truly the highest academic position to which a faculty member can be appointed.

Universities, as we know them, carry with them many of the symbols

JOYCE J. FITZPATRICK, PhD, RN, FAAN, is dean of Nursing, and Elizabeth Brooks Ford Professor of Nursing at Frances Payne Bolton School of Nursing, Case Western Reserve University, Cleveland, OH. This article is an edited version of a speech presented at the University of Pittsburgh School of Nursing 50th Anniversary Program, May 14, 1990. M. ELIZABETH CARNEGIE, DPA, RN, FAAN, is Distinguished Visiting Professor, Indiana University School of Nursing.

from the Middle Ages. For example, much of the activity that surrounds our commencement exercises: the robes, the caps, and the hoods, as well as the processions and academic degrees, derive from our early beginnings. Many of our titles—doctors, masters, professors, donors—date from the early university days.

The hallmarks of the early university were twofold: a place where students from all over were received to study in freedom; and a guild or club, the organizational structure which became the university.

Universities were founded upon the concept of freedom: freedom of assembly and freedom of inquiry. Cardinal Newman, in his classic work on the idea of the university published in the mid-19th century, viewed the university as a "place of teaching universal knowledge." While universities have frequently enjoyed a close relationship to both church and state, there has existed a clear and predominant value for freedom. The endowed chair makes that possible and preserves the freedom of inquiry that is so necessary to the university.

Chair as Symbol of Status

In the early beginnings of the universities, a chair was a rare article of furniture and, therefore, highly prized. The commoners sat on three-legged stools or benches, and the gentry used cushions. Only the very distinguished, no-

Reprinted from *Nursing Outlook* Sept/Oct 1991, Vol. 39, No. 5. Copyright © 1991 American Journal of Nursing Company. Reprinted by permission of Mosby, Inc. A Harcourt Health Sciences Company.

tably monarchs and high churchmen, used chairs. Thus, when a worthy faculty member was accorded the university rank of Professor, he also received an actual chair as a symbol of his high status. These chairs were most often provided by donors, who at first provided actual chairs for the professors to sit upon. As the universities developed, so also did the method of support of professors change. Chairs were initially provided as articles of furniture, and later became supported by endowment funds committed by a donor. Today, an endowed chair connotes a significant fund established and invested to support the educational pursuits of a highly acclaimed educator/researcher or scientist. The endowed chair honors the person for whom it is named, often the donor, and the Professor.

It might also be interesting to note here the history of the other type of major endowments in universities, i.e., named scholarships which also honor the donor and the student recipient. In the early days of universities, students paid the teacher in cash or goods for the instruction they received. In fact, at Case Western Reserve University, founded in 1826, archival records show that payments had been made in beef and other consumables. In the early days, poor students were also supported by Chests. Here, benefactors deposited money in an iron chest from which loans were granted to destitute and deserving students. Today, we have endowed scholarships.

Well, enough of the early ages of universities. What relevance does this have for nursing education and, particularly, for nursing today, as we struggle to become full participating members of the academic communities?

Nursing is a relatively new discipline in academia. Thus, our establishment of endowed chairs in nursing has been relatively recent. As of 1990, we have approximately 50 endowed chairs in nursing in this country. Only 11 of those were established before 1980. Therefore, approximately 40 endowed chairs in nursing have been established in the past decade, a remarkable accomplishment for academic nursing, and a development which is so critical for our future academic and scientific endeavors.

The general rule of thumb at Case Western University, for example, is that

there should be an endowed professorship, an endowed chair, for each faculty member at the full professor rank. We are in the very fortunate position in our School of Nursing now to have twice as many endowed chairs—six—as full professors.

Advantages of Endowed Chairs

What are the advantages of endowed chairs? While there are several advantages that I'd like to highlight, I first want to emphasize the most critical ele-

ment, i.e., the freedom of inquiry, the true sense of our university foundation that is so important to our academic and professional future. The endowment funds from a named professorship support the faculty member to do his or her research. We can encourage a freedom of scholarship that is not tied to government research funds.

Particularly now, in developing the discipline of nursing, we must have some senior scholars who have this freedom to contemplate our scientific course. In the past two years, our nursing research has expanded considerably, and our conceptualization of the discipline has developed from some early theory statements in the 1960s to sophisticated theoretical developments today.

The University's establishment of an endowed chair represents the ultimate form of institutional legitimization for the discipline and provides formal authority for the researcher who occupies the chair. An endowed chair provides the research opportunities to develop high visibility for the respective discipline, to advance a focused research program, and to create an environment for socializing novice faculty members. Persons who occupy endowed chairs may serve as "magnets" to attract additional funding and other scholars, in-

cluding students and faculty. To be named to an endowed professorship is truly one of the highest academic honors that one can receive. It is important that we continue to support this development in schools of nursing.

As relative newcomers to academia, nurse researchers are faced with the dual challenge of establishing the legitimacy of their discipline and their performance as scientists. The funding of endowed research chairs in nursing can provide the necessary freedom for our

---

Nursing is a relatively new discipline in academia and the establishment of endowed chairs in nursing has been recent: Of the approximately 50 endowed chairs in nursing, only 11 were established before 1980.

---

nurse researchers' scientific pursuits. The endowed chair is a symbol that is widely recognized by the academic community as a means of facilitating research, ensuring quality, promoting the socialization of upcoming scientists, and rewarding demonstrated commitment and scholarly productivity.

A fully endowed chair (at our university, approximately $1 million to $1.25 million) provides annual income for a faculty position held by an accomplished scholar in a particular field of study. The principal in an endowment fund is left untouched and only the income generated by the principal is used annually.

To give you some perspective on where we are and where we need to go, it should be noted that, prior to 1980, there were only 11 endowed professorships in nursing, nationally. At that same time, the Medical School at Case Western Reserve University had 22 endowed chairs, twice the number that were endowed in nursing, nationally. It is important for us, as nurses, to become more fully integrated within our universities.

The First Endowed Chair in Nursing

As a summary, it may be of interest to share some of the highlights of the establishment of the *first* endowed chair in nursing, at the University of Virginia in 1928—a chair endowed not by one philanthropic donor, as most chairs are given by one donor, but rather a chair endowed by hundreds of nurses, many members of the Virginia Nurses Association and many alumni of the various Virginia schools of nursing. Under the leadership of one nurse, Agnes Dillon Randolph, at the 23rd Annual State Nurses Convention, the members agreed to assume the task of raising the $50,000 necessary for the chair and to name it in honor of Virginia's pioneer nurse Sadie Heath-Cabaniss. They began a campaign in which no donation was considered too small. Nurses reached deeply into their own limited resources and made generous contributions. The average annual salary of a nurse then was $1,000 per year. These nurses were asked to commit $5 a year for 2 years. At today's

cation of (Southern) nurses which would free them and open to them wider doors of opportunity...

Endowed chairs in nursing are about freedom and opportunity for our scholarship, our research and our profession.

On Filling Endowed Chairs in Nursing
M. Elizabeth Carnegie

How is the chairholder selected? What does the holder of a chair do? What is the average salary or salary range? These are a few of the many questions asked by those not familiar with the concept of an endowed chair. Endowed chairs have a long tradition, having been in existence for nearly 500 years. According to materials in the Duke University Archives in Durham, North Carolina, one of the earliest named professorships, or chairs, in the

funds. The state then matches that total, making the minimum chair endowment $1 million.[1]

The State of Tennessee has appropriated $43 million for 80 chairs of Excellence, 76 of which have been endowed with more than $31.3 million from private sources. The chairholder's salary, moving expenses, travel, staff, and office expenses are paid for from interest accrued from the endowment. A chairholder's salary in Tennessee may range from $60,000 to $90,000 for a 12-month contract, considerably higher than salaries of other faculty members. The goal is to find national scholars in any field who will bolster a school's reputation and help attract top faculty and graduate students to the particular field. The chair of Excellence in Nursing at Memphis State University (MSU) was endowed in 1988 with $1 million by William A. and Ruth F. Loewenberg. Mr. Loewenberg is a Memphis businessman and philanthropist.[1] In 1990, the Loewenbergs endowed the School of Nursing at MSU.

To provide basic information on endowed chairs in nursing, in 1984 Fitzpatrick surveyed schools of nursing in universities. At that time 21 endowed chairs in nursing were identified and reported in terms of the date of initial endowment, the amount of the endowment, the focus, and the name. Many more have been established since then and some have more than one chair, e.g. Emory University Neil Hodgson Woodruff School of Nursing in Atlanta, Georgia, has two $1 million endowments, the first was endowed by the Independence Foundation in Philadelphia as part of its commitment to impact the nursing shortage in the United States and is currently occupied by Ora Strickland, PhD, RN, FAAN.

According to Fitzpatrick, "an endowed chair establishes a permanent professorship in the academic structure of the university. These professorships are awarded to highly acclaimed individuals who have made significant contributions to scholarship in the designated area. The endowed professorship is the most prestigious faculty position in a university. In addition, it provides distinction and recognition to the donor and the university."[2]

Although the first endowed chair in nursing was in 1928 at the University of

---

The endowed professorship, or chair, is the most prestigious faculty position in a university. In addition, it provides distinction and recognition to the donor and the university.

---

rates, the nurse with an annual salary of $25,000 would be asked to commit $125 a year. To endow a chair today at a million and a quarter, with the average gift of $125, would require 10,000 such contributions. While that may seem like a monumental task, it is also one that is possible to accomplish.

We have many lessons to learn from our great nursing leaders. The most important of which is to create change, it requires a great leader. The fate of nursing education and scholarship is truly in all of our hands as, individually and collectively, we provide leadership for our profession.

The words of Agnes Dillon Randolph, who led the effort in establishing the first chair in nursing at the University of Virginia, should remind us all how far we have come:

I was trained...in a small training school, dominated by the old aristocratic traditions. I pledged myself then to make some contribution to the edu-

United States was created for Harvard University in 1816 by Abriel Smith, a Boston merchant.

Duke University in Durham, North Carolina, bears special witness to its intellectual commitment through its program of distinguished professorships, or named chairs. Appointment to a named chair is the highest honor the University can bestow upon a member of its faculty, irrespective of field.

Memphis State University in Memphis, Tennessee, has 18 Chairs of Excellence, part of a multimillion-dollar statewide program begun by Governor Lamar Alexander's 1984 better schools program. The chair's plan was introduced by State Representative John Bragg who wanted a program that could sustain itself with one-time funding through endowments. Under Tennessee's endowment formula, a private source puts up a minimum of $250,000 which in turn is matched by university funds or reallocation of university

Virginia School of Nursing, the movement toward endowed chairs in nursing is fairly recent.[3,4] Chairs are usually named after their donors but, in some cases, a chair is named in honor of a person who has made a significant contribution to the nursing profession. For example, the Alumni Association of Teachers College, Columbia University, New York, raised money to endow a chair named in honor of Isabel Stewart. The chair at Tuskegee University in Alabama is named for Mary Starke Harper, an alumnus; the one at Howard University College of Nursing in Washington, D.C. will be named The M. Elizabeth Carnegie Chair. The University of Iowa College of Nursing in Iowa City has plans for establishing "an endowed chair to honor a distinguished minority alumnus."[5]

Occupying Endowed Chairs

In 1978, I took early retirement from the editorship of *Nursing Research* after 25 years on the editorial staff of the American Journal of Nursing Company in New York. Before then, I had been dean of two baccalaureate nursing programs. In the 12 years since my retirement, I have held visiting distinguished professorships at six universities including the current one at Indiana University and have occupied two endowed chairs—one at Adelphi University, Garden City, New York; the other at Memphis State University, Memphis, Tennessee. Both were firsts for nursing in those universities.

Adelphi University. The Chair in Nursing at Adelphi University was endowed in 1985 by Dr. James Bender and named in honor of his wife, Vera E. Bender who is a nurse. Upon invitation of the administration and faculty, I became the first occupant of the chair for the academic year, 1987–1988. Because this was to be a new experience for me, I sought advice from John Hope Franklin, an internationally known historian who had held the James E. Duke Chair at Duke University for a number of years.

Memphis State University. Again, I was the first to occupy the Loewenberg Chair of Excellence at Memphis State University School of Nursing for the academic year, 1989–1990. Having held the Chair at Adelphi University, I was able to share my experiences with the faculty

and suggest how I might be of service to them. As a consequence, my activities fell into the following categories: lectures to 16 different classes plus a university- and community-wide lecture during Black History Month; faculty seminar on writing; editorial assistance to faculty; individual conferences with faculty and students, including those from other departments and schools in the university; community activities; and the conduct of my own research, which was historical in nature.

My experiences at Memphis State University were similar to those at Adelphi with the addition of the writing seminar for faculty, community activities, and conduct of my own research. The major objective of the writing seminar was to have each faculty prepare a paper for possible publication in a scholarly journal. Whereas I had no involvement in the community where Adelphi is located, I could not fill all the speaking engagements requested of me in Memphis and the surrounding areas. This may have been due to the extensive press coverage of my occupying the Loewenberg Chair of Excellence in Nursing.

As for the conduct of my own research, I compiled a 1991 historical calendar for the National League for Nursing on the 23 baccalaureate and higher degree nursing programs at historically Black colleges and universities in the United States and started writing the second edition of my book, *The Path We Tread: Blacks in Nursing, 1854–1990.* Also, at the request of the editor of the *American Nurse,* my article, "Blacks in Nursing: An Update," appeared in the February 1990 issue. This I wrote while at Memphis State University.

While I appreciate the favorable comments from faculty and students on my contributions at Adelphi and Memphis

State, it was a two-way street; that is, I also learned and grew from the experience of occupying an endowed chair. Although I did not carry a teaching load in either university, I enjoyed all the rights and privileges of a faculty member.

Chairholder an Inspiring Presence

The very presence of a chairholder sometimes inspires others to expand their interests, including doing research, writing for publication, and even developing a desire to further their education. In other words, he or

> *The very presence of a chairholder sometimes inspires others to expand their interests. Scholars do not operate in a vacuum. Availability of other faculty with expertise in related areas offer opportunities for cross-fertilization and collaboration.*

she serves as a role model to students and faculty and is available to advise less experienced faculty members in teaching and research.

It is a well-known fact that scholars do not operate in a vacuum. Availability of other faculty with expertise in the same or related area offers a tremendous opportunity for cross-fertilization and collaboration on selected educational and research projects.

Hopefully, my activities in these two chairs at Adelphi and Memphis State Universities will serve as a guide for others and answer some questions. They were both rewarding experiences.

REFERENCES

1. Energetic author fills MSU Chair in nursing; endowment boosts schools, *The Commercial Appeal* (Memphis, TN) Oct.29, 1989, pp. B 1,2.
2. Fitzpatrick J.K. Endowed chairs in nursing: state of the art, *J.Prof.Nurs.* 1:145–147, May-June 1985.
3. ____. Endowed chairs in nursing: an update, *J.Prof.Nurs.* 2:261–262, July-Aug. 1986.
4. ____. Endowed chairs in nursing: 1988 update, *J.Prof.Nurs.* 5:23–24, Jan-Feb. 1989.
5. Felton, G. Nursing and the academic enterprise: a covenant with quality, In *The Nursing Profession; Turning points* ed by N.L. Chaska. St. Louis, C.V. Mosby Co., 1990.

Appendix D

Fundraising Articles

Primer for Philanthropy

The ABCs of Fundraising

Sandra S. Deller, BA

Joyce J. Fitzpatrick
PhD, RN, MBA, FAAN

A- a broad-based development program
B- background research and preparation
C- cultivation and solicitation
= DOLLARS

Development is a people business. Philanthropy is the application of interpersonal skills, leadership, management, and listening skills. Concepts are as basic as the ABCs. It is the application and individualization that translate to donor involvement and, subsequently, dollars. This "primer" addresses key components of a successful program of fundraising, including annual funds, major gifts, and endowments, and presents strategies that have been proven effective.

The Annual Fund

Development includes a broad-based program beginning with a well developed annual fund as foundation. The Annual Fund is a yearly campaign for unrestricted operating dollars. Most often, it is this vehicle that provides an opportunity to become close to potential donors. Individuals who have been consistent donors, or those who increase or decrease support, should receive special attention.

Response to the Annual Fund drive is an indicator of your constituents' interests and commitment. If the Annual Fund is solicited by direct mail and meets with a good response rate, it indicates a very invested group of alumni/ae and friends; however, direct mail is generally the least effective form of solicitation. The high volume of unsolicited appeals is staggering and competition is fierce. A combination of direct mail and telemarketing is more effective. Phone contact (telemarketing) elicits more personal information about supporters. Most effective is the combination of some direct solicitation, telemarketing, and direct mail. The mechanism is determined by the potential of the donor. If an individual has been a regular donor over several years, consider the advantage of a personal visit in generating increased support. Donor lists should be segmented according to giving potential and staff resources. The time commitment for individual visits will be well worth the effort, both in immediate gains and in building knowledge of the individual, developing relationships, and set-ting the stage for more significant future contributions.

There is a plethora of gift options suitable for an Annual Fund. These include the following:

• Anniversary Gifts—anniversary or reunion gifts are the easiest to secure. The request

The time commitment for individual visits will be well worth the effort, both in immediate gains and in building knowledge of the individual, developing relationships, and setting the stage for more significant future contributions.

▲ ▲ ▲

is based on the year of graduation with special attention to 5-year periods.

• Challenge Gifts—an immediate way to increase your annual fund revenue is to ask one of the school's closest friends and donors to issue a challenge to his or her classmates. The ratio can be a $1-per-$1 basis with a limit, or require that for every $1 there would be a $2 match from donors.

• Gift Clubs—and honor rolls are lists that group names according to categories of support, such as the Dean's Club or President's Society, or that could be named for a founder or outstanding alumnus. These lists are published and provide an incentive for classmates to be included in similar clubs or societies for peer recognition.

Reprinted from *Nursing Leadership Forum*, Fall 1998, Vol. 3, No. 3. Copyright © 1997. Reprinted by permission of Springer Publishing Company.

▲ ▲ ▲

If the potential of the

prospect is great enough,

no source should be left

unexplored in preparing for

the solicitation.

▲ ▲ ▲

• Celebrate Special Occasions—be certain to be opportunistic in using any special event or anniversary to pitch a special gift to the Annual Fund that might be a larger gift than usual, what is referred to as a "stretch gift."

Volumes have been written about conducting successful Annual Fund campaigns and the pros and cons of various appeals and methodology. The role of the Annual Fund is a critical first stage for development.

Major Gifts

The definition of a major gift depends upon the organization. For some, the largest gifts are in the $5,000-to-$10,000 range; for others, the threshold is $25,000 or even $100,000. Regardless of the range, the secrets to a major gift are relationships and follow-up. Major gifts involve 95% cultivation and 5% solicitation. Look first to those closest to the school or organization such as trustees, chairs of committees, current or emeriti faculty, or active alumni/ae: "the insiders." These individuals will often have suggestions for major gift prospects, how much the prospect might be willing to give, the most effective approach, or which project(s) would interest the prospect. Like the Annual Fund, prospects for major gifts should be segmented.

Additionally, the group of donors who have made larger or regular contributions to the Annual Fund, a building fund or a special project should be asked to join "the insiders" by taking

a leadership role in fundraising. After they have made a commitment, they can be asked to identify others: alumni/ae, colleagues or friends who might be interested in the campaign or project.

A third tier of prospects, those who have given smaller gifts or whose giving has been sporadic, should be contacted. Expanding contacts increases the prospect base and potential support. Consider any legacies of the school; generations of family involvement can lead to a mega gift. Tour facilities and research names on existing plaques, consulting archival donor lists for recognition. Tributes are valuable resources.

Major gifts require a customized, individual approach. Not all contacts will result in a gift, but at the very least they will lay the fundraising foundation. Additionally, you are gathering important data about how the school or organization is perceived. This, too, can be helpful in developing prospective contacts related to initiatives and may even provide valuable insights about enhancing current programs and developing new projects. With continued contact and cultivation, future development is facilitated.

Endowment

It is important to maintain a balance between outright (unrestricted) and endowment gifts. Endowment is a legacy for the school as well as the donor. Wise investment of the principal and allocation of a percentage of the interest annually to be spent for the donor's intention guarantee its permanence. The percentage varies among institutions but often is around 5%. The remaining interest is returned to the principal to ensure its future growth and perpetuity. There is a broad range of endowment gift opportunities, including student support, faculty support or recognition, capital projects (buildings or renovations), programs, research, lectures, library funds and special awards. There is usually a minimum cost to establish an endowment fund; often, however, there is some allowance for individuals to make a pledge with payments over time, typically 3 to 5 years. Many donors find endowment giving very appealing, especially attaching the family name for perpetuity as an honor or memorial.

The named endowment fund provides an excellent opportunity to communicate with donors. Appropriate acknowledgment of all gifts is important but especially endowment giving,

as recognition was probably a motivator for the gift. Some tangible remembrance, such as a plaque with the family name prominently displayed, a description of the fund's purpose and the date of its establishment, is always welcomed. Also, include endowment donors in publications, honor rolls, or lists of supporters.

Research

Research is the basis for determining the who, what, and when for fundraising—the resources. While a research department is extremely valuable, much can be accomplished with the proper focus on priority prospects. Information that can provide important clues to a donor's capacity or propensity to contribute includes personal information, such as date of birth, marital status, number of children, home and business addresses, education, career or any financial information on the prospect's company, including compensation and stock options. All of this information is very valuable in determining a feasible gift range. With public companies, information is easy to ascertain from annual reports and income tax returns. Private companies require more thorough research. Additional areas that assist with insights are other relationships with the school, especially legacies, student offices, associations, and sports activities. Information on community activities is helpful particularly if the individual or spouse is a trustee or significant donor. Any information about the prospect's philanthropy will be helpful in targeting how much to request. If the potential of the prospect is great enough, no source should be left unexplored in preparing for the solicitation. Friends, colleagues and faculty, including emeriti faculty, should be consulted as they often have personal information about the prospect. Gathering background information can make the critical difference in the outcome of your solicitation.

Securing the Appointment

As simple as it sounds, this sometimes proves to be the most difficult. Without a face-to-face meeting, cultivation and solicitation cannot occur. As with other fundraising initiatives, there are many methods and styles used to schedule appointments. Some prefer to make the call themselves; others like to have an assistant make the contact. Development personnel should apply the method that is optimal for the staff and school. Sometimes it is effective to prepare the prospect for the call by first sending an introductory letter. If there is an "insider" who is close to the individual, it might be desirable for that person to secure the appointment. A disadvantage of employing this method is the timeliness and availability of the volunteer caller.

With a busy executive, an assistant who is a "gate keeper" can be a formidable obstacle. Engage the assistant and enlist him or her to help schedule the appointment. An alternative method is to assume a familiarity with the executive by using his/her first name. Timing can facilitate access, e.g., calling early in the morning, at lunchtime, or after regular hours can sometimes provide direct contact to the prospect. If this fails, a call to the executive's home might be considered.

As a last resort, leave a compelling message on an answering machine, send a fax, or use e-mail. If the message on the machine is informal, be informal in your approach. Try a teaser to get a response: "*I am calling from the president's* or *dean's office*" or "*your friend, George, suggested we talk.*" Always maintain control by stating when you will be calling back to schedule the appointment.

Another question that arises is how much information to provide the prospect. Ideally, give only enough information to secure the appointment. Providing too much information or too many details can lead the individual to restrict the conversation to only phone contact or conclude that the information provided was sufficient and there is no need for a personal meeting.

Like so much of development, securing the appointment requires a sensitivity to the prospect. Does the individual sound busy? If so, do not proceed with the appointment request as it will probably not be successful. The most effective callers are those individuals who can immediately engage the individual. Instead, ask when would be a good time to call back. Positive expectations can elicit positive responses. After the appointment is arranged, confirm it in writing to make certain that all parties have the correct information.

Cultivation

The initial step in cultivation is to select the most appropriate individual(s) to meet with the prospect. Past history and relationships are key factors. In some cases, it will be the dean,

organization CEO, department chair or faculty member. Additionally, a team comprising a development professional, volunteer, dean or faculty member, or some combination of these individuals, could make the approach. Each situation requires a unique approach and there is no "right" formula.

Cultivation entails establishing or strengthening the individual's interest or involvement in the school or project. It normally involves several meetings with the individual and/or spouse, including special activities designed to increase their affiliation with the school. Each meeting should have a specific goal. The number of meetings should be determined by the response and feedback of the individual prospect.

The first visit with a new prospect is a discovery mission. It is essential to find out how the school is perceived and its value to the prospect's career or personal life. Information the prospect volunteers about relationships, morals, attitudes, and activities can provide important clues in formulating the next step in the cultivation. If the meeting is in the prospect's home or office, take careful note of the surroundings and furnishing styles. These appointments reveal personality; look for items of commonality such as photographs of children or a hobby. These serve as great ice breakers for conversation. Body language and posture, beginning with the handshake, help define personality traits, style, and chemistry with the development team. Specifically, you are trying to discover what will motivate the prospect to make a gift. Why give and why now? What benefits can giving to the school or project present for the donor? People give for a variety of reasons, for example, recognition, immortality, to perpetuate their own beliefs or values, to belong, out of a sense of responsibility, or to ameliorate guilt.

The most effective contacts are usually those in which the prospect does most of the talking, and the development team, the listening. A few well-placed, open-ended questions, attentive listening, and keen observations can accelerate cultivation.

Solicitation

With sufficient research and cultivation, the solicitation can proceed. Strategies should be set for the solicitation and the lead solicitor selected in advance. It is usually advisable not to solicit solo; two heads and ears are better than one.

▲ ▲ ▲

The first visit with a new prospect is a discovery mission.

▲ ▲ ▲

Sometimes, rehearsing possible scenarios provides a level of comfort and can help prepare the team to address objections. A positive mind set should be maintained throughout the call. The setting should be comfortable for the prospect, e.g., breakfast, lunch or meetings in the home or office. A predetermined time limit should be followed. As with earlier contacts, the individual's temperament affects the solicitation climate. Engage the prospect in conversation related to an item from earlier discussions or the latest shared experience, either business or personal.

When appropriate, the conversation should segue into the solicitation. Again, there is no "right" way to ask. The request must be clear and unequivocal. Ask for the order. Whatever the style or format, the request must be tied to the purpose, cost and, if applicable, a time limit. It can be straightforward, "*as one of our closest friends, we would like you to consider a gift to* ___ *of $* ___ *to support* ___." Another approach could be, "*we know you (e.g., Joan) are committed to the School - how do you want to be identified in this campaign?*" or "*it seems like this project is something you care about, you can help us with a gift of $* ___ *to help initiate this program.*" If a lighter approach is called for, "*Joan, we appreciate your generous annual fund gift and wondered if you would consider adding a couple more zeros for this important project.*" If a volunteer is present, it can be effective for the volunteer to suggest, "*Joan, please join me in supporting this project with a gift of $* ___." Sometimes, the volunteer can be a little uncomfortable soliciting a friend. Proper coaching of the volunteer, with a lead-in from the development professional, can often achieve the desired results.

Successful solicitations are not dependent upon the most articulate request; rather, they

Too often, the temptation is to keep talking, but silence on the part of those making the request is important.

▲ ▲ ▲

depend on the rationale for the gift, matching of gift needs, and sincerity of the solicitor. After the proposal, the solicitation team should remain silent and allow the prospect to respond. Too often, the temptation is to keep talking, but silence on the part of those making the request is important. Based on the response, the follow-up, either in the form of a proposal or additional information, should be discussed. If a commitment is made, details, such as pledge forms, should be completed. Affirm the importance of the donor's support.

If the decision is delayed, the solicitor should call in a few weeks to a month to see if the timing is better. A "no" is *not* always a "no" in fundraising and "no" does *not* mean "never." The old sales adage, "a sale begins with the first refusal," often holds true. Timing is a key ingredient; also, there may be another need of the school that is more closely aligned to the prospect's priorities. Above all, persistence does pay. Meetings should always end on a positive note. At the very least, it was a public relations call for the school or organization. A successful solicitation team warrants congratulations and commences the stewardship process.

Stewardship

An important caveat to remember in fundraising is that a donor can never be thanked too often or by too many people. The solicitation team should send a note; the dean, lead faculty or volunteer should send another note. If appropriate, the president should add an acknowledgment, too. The donor's name should be included on recognition lists (if not anonymous) and the donor and family should be invited to all significant activities. By being as inclusive as possible, the relationship will be strengthened.

If the donor lives out of town, the development staff or primary contact should maintain the relationship and visit when possible. Visits by faculty or volunteers will keep ties strong. Sending information related to the donor's area of interest and news items also maintains contact. Donors should feel like "insiders" and be treated accordingly. Regular reports should be sent to the donors detailing the use of their funds. Reports should include information on the growth of their fund and market value, the use of their fund, and the program or project that the fund benefits. If the fund is a scholarship fund, it is helpful to send information about the student award recipients, such as their grades, accomplishments, major, and hometown. When possible, a meeting should be arranged so the donor's philanthropy is tangible. Students can be the best salespeople for additional gifts. Often, lifelong relationships are developed through these meetings. If a meeting is not possible, student recipients should be asked to send the donor a thank-you note and tell the donor a little about themselves and their educational experiences, future professional goals, and what the support means to them. Special annual events to recognize significant donors with the board, president, dean and key faculty present, also serve to enhance stewardship and reinforce that the donor and other attendees are truly the school's best friends.

Cultivation, solicitation and stewardship are all a continuum, that is, critical to prospecting for the annual fund, major gifts, and endowments. Today's donors are tomorrow's legacies and can benefit the school in countless ways. It is a win-win situation; the donor feels proud to be part of a quality institution and the school gains support to accomplish its mission.

▲ ▲ ▲

Sandra S. Deller, BA, is Special Assistant to the Vice President and Director of Major Gifts, Case Western Reserve University. Xavier University Fundraising professional for over 17 years.

Joyce J. Fitzpatrick, PhD, RN, MBA, FAAN, is a visiting scholar at New York University, Divisions of Nursing, New York, NY.

▲

Twelve Principles of Successful Fund-Raising

Joyce J. Fitzpatrick,
PhD, MBA, RN, FAAN

Health profession schools traditionally have been dependent upon public support for academic programs. This article is focused on generating private support from a range of sources. Attention will be paid to the structures and the processes to generate new avenues of private support for academic programs. Successful examples that have been used in the last 10 years at Case Western Reserve University are given to highlight the principles addressed.

The goal of philanthropy is to improve the human condition. Two of our noblest institutions, hospitals and universities, have been built upon philanthropy and have evolved through numerous kinds of gift-giving programs. It is of interest to note that philanthropy increases as the economy declines. It is an important foundation of philanthropy to note that people give to people. Thus, the personal approach can make the difference in

any effort to generate support for academic programs. The art of asking involves the *right* program, the *right* purpose, and the *right* amount.

Individuals may give for a variety of reasons: They want to maintain their own immortality; they want to live in perpetuity; they want to perpetuate their own beliefs; they want to belong to something; they want recognition; or they want to alleviate ills. For many people, giving is based on a sense of duty, a belief that one should support the future generations. On a related note, as educators it is important for us to instill in our students the sense of responsibility and duty that they must give to the students who come after them.

The following 12 principles are presented as a basis for fund-raising activities.

Principle 1: Volunteers are an important resource in generating private support.
Structures that we have put in place to increase the activities of volunteers include a formal advisory committee and campaign/development committee structures with subcommittees. For example, we have volunteers assisting with our recruitment activity for students for the School of Nursing. We have volunteers participating on various campaign committees. We have a very structured volunteer organization among our alumni. We have many different committees participating, but the important point is that the volunteers have a lot of the responsibility for generating support for our programs. In the last decade, alumni giving has increased by approximately 70%; we could not have done that without our volunteer structure. Peer solicitation is what makes the difference. If you are asked to support the Alumni Association by a classmate who graduated in the same year, then you are more likely to participate in that activity. We use our volunteer structure for all of our fund-raising activities. Each of our six endowed chairs that we have generated in the last 10 years can be traced to a volunteer who had been actively involved in the solicitation.

▲ ▲ ▲

People give to people.
Thus, the personal
approach can make the
difference in any effort to
generate support for
academic programs.

▲ ▲ ▲

Principle 2: Public and private support are often intertwined.
In a private institution you find most clearly the relationship between public and private support. A few examples are relevant here. One is the specific activity of Congresswoman Frances Payne Bolton, who as a private citizen endowed our School of Nursing, then became a Representative of Congress and was very active in the public funding not just of nursing at Case Western Reserve University but of nursing nationally. It is very important to find ways to link private funding with public funding. We have discovered that there most often are links that can be developed. We have recently created a new primary health care center as a part of our faculty practice in the School of Nursing. Because of the private support that we were able to generate for this particular project, we also were able to secure a federal grant to support activities of the center.

Principle 3: Maintain and nurture the relationships that you develop.
Every week we talk about our activities in fund-raising and friend-raising. Once you develop a circle of friends, it is important to support every link in the circle. Keep everybody involved in the development activities at all times. One

▲ ▲ ▲

For academic institutions

and for many other private

institutions, endowment is

the foundation for all of the

other development activity.

Endowment funding is an

investment in the future.

▲ ▲ ▲

example of continued involvement is as follows. In 1988, we completed a $5 million campaign. There were key volunteers involved in the committee structure; we asked them to stay on for the next campaign committee, and gave them responsibility as consultants to the new committee. Thus, we try to nurture the relationships that we develop and keep volunteers involved over time.

Principle 4: It is important to be successful in your goal.

In the campaign that we completed in June 1994, we struggled with identifying a campaign goal. Our 1988 campaign goal for the School of Nursing was $5 million and was the most we had ever raised in a campaign for the school. So we needed to be cautious. At the same time, we had uncovered a great deal of potential, so we knew that we had to be somewhere beyond $5 million, but realistic in setting a goal. Most important, we needed to set a goal that we could achieve. We set a goal of $15 million, knowing that we could achieve $15 million. The struggle was to set the goal at $15 million and not at $25 million. Over the five-year campaign, we raised $26 million. We were able to boast that we went $11 million over our goal, whereas, if we had set it at $25 million, we would only be $1 million

over goal. It is more impressive to be $11 million over goal than to be $1 million over. The most important point is to set a goal that you know you can achieve; everyone wants to support a winner. Create the system so you can win.

During the campaign that closed in 1994, we raised $7 million from corporations. Prior to this campaign, that is, prior to 1989, we had raised more than $100,000 from any corporation in any 1 year. We focused on generating foundation support and were able to raise close to $9 million from foundations. Previous to 1989, we had not had a very strong showing in foundation funding. Prior to this 1989-1994 campaign, most of our support had been from individuals.

Principle 5: Development requires a long-term perspective.

It is important to plant the seeds for one's successors. It takes time to identify the relationships that fit with the particular development goals. Of course, for academic institutions and for many other private institutions, endowment is the foundation for all of the other development activity. Endowment funding is an investment in the future.

In academic institutions, an endowed chair represents the ultimate form of an institutional legitimization of disciplines. Endowed chairs were noted as early as 1449. An endowed chair provides funding support for scholarly pursuits at the highest academic level. It is interesting to note that in 1928 the first endowed chair in nursing was committed by the nurses themselves. Many of the individuals who contributed were alumni of the University of Virginia, and many of them were not. They were all members of the Virginia Nurses' Association. It was several years before any others were endowed. Endowed chairs provide an opportunity for high visibility for both the professor and the school.

What follows is a description of some general aspects of philanthropy in the United States. These figures can be traced each year. If increases in contributions over the last 5 years are traced, there is an approximately 5.5% or 6% increase annually in the contributions. If you think about approximately $124.3 billion being given privately to support programs, it seems that many schools are not getting a fair share of that $124.3 billion. Individual giving accounts for 89% of every dollar given. This is important because, in terms of long-term development activity, it

really makes sense to focus on individuals. Although it may be easier to write foundation proposals or corporate proposals, the greater payoff is in individual support. In 1992, $7.78 billion were given in individual bequests alone. Foundation grants were only $8 billion in 1992. Corporate giving was only $6 billion. Individual giving accounts for most of the private support, close to 9 cents out of 10. Yet it requires a lot more activity and more of a long-term perspective, particularly with new alumni because it takes them a while to accumulate resources. In 1992, gifts to education were $14 billion and gifts to human services were $111 billion.

The following is an example used in our previous two campaigns. Individuals were offered the opportunity to name scholars in the academic programs. The students know who' their sponsor is, and the donors know who their students are. Interactions between donor and students are encouraged. Our expectation is that this relationship will continue over the years. We hope we are building in the responsibility to the students so that they know that they have been supported by an individual in their academic career and they will feel some responsibility to suport future students.

Principle 6: It matters whom you know.

It is important to nurture relationships and to ' try to know everybody that you possibly can. For example, we found that we often had physicians telling us that nurses were not like they used to be and if we prepared them better, everything would be like it used to be. So we said, "OK, you can help, folks. Here is how you can do it, you can help us, you can give us some money, we will prepare them differently and you can be involved." We set up a physicians' advisory committee, but we also set up a scholarship fund. We did get all of our friends to participate and were able to raise close to $250,000 from physicians who wanted to support nursing education, and most important, who wanted to be involved in some way. The way they were involved is through an advisory committee that recommended students to us. We have a number of students who were recommended by physicians in the community because they knew more about our program. We sent our physician friends a lot of literature about our programs. By the way of involvement, we did set up a separate physicians' scholarship . fund and we monitor that yearly; we report to them yearly about whom they are supporting and what kind of support they are providing. That circle of friends we knew in the physician community was extremely important to us in raising the money. We did presentations at medical staff meetings in community hospitals and we made house calls to physicians' offices to tell them about the program. We approached banks and businesses where we knew that somebody happened to know a nurse. We involved corporate executives who had a particular interest in health care. We have started involving people in public policy discussions with the expectation that we will extend our network.

Principle 7: Collaboration with other academic programs provides a foundation.

In our community and in our university, there is no way we could have initiated the programs and generated the support we have without the collaboration of academic programs. We have a strong collaborative activity around certain academic programs, but it is very clear that that collaboration was a key to our success both in terms of program planning and in terms of product support. An example of our collaboration is our previously mentioned Nursing Health Center, which is a primary health care and birthing service developed in an underserved area. Here we have been able to generate approximately $1 million in private foundation support. Important, collaboration with the School of Medicine was required to launch this project because every time we came up against some regulatory barriers to advanced nursing practice, the phone calls about what was happening did not come to the School of Nursing, they came to the School of Medicine. So we require that we be involved in communication with colleagues, particularly in the School of Medicine.

Principle 8: Take risks.

Almost all the programs that we have launched in the last 8 years have been launched through outside funding. Almost all of them have involved some degree of risk. For example, we recently began an acute care pediatric nurse practitioner program in collaboration with two hospitals in the community. We have discovered that there are questions about certification of graduates from this program. We have to be involved in setting the standards at the national level to clarify the "gray area" of certification.

Principle 9: Involve faculty at all levels.

I almost never can speak as well about the academic programs as the faculty. It is very typical to have the key faculty members present the case for funding because, although it is important for me to be there as the academic administrator, it is more important to have someone there who can answer the questions. We have found that it is most important to have the expertise of the faculty in all of our efforts to generate academic program support.

Principle 10: Alumni are forever.

We treat our alumni as if they are forever because we know they are key to our outreach efforts, as well as to our annual fund efforts which serve as the base for our overall development. We have many programs orchestrated to keep our alumni active at all levels.

Principle 11: You have to spend money to make money.

Sometimes this is particularly difficult if you do not already have a lot of money to spend. When I received the first commitment for the $5 million campaign that we launched in 1983, we turned a few faculty positions into staff positions for development. It was important to invest in that campaign in order to be successful. Also, in development it is expected that expenses will be justified. In the campaign completed in 1994, the School of Nursing had the lowest investment in our development costs; fewer than 10 cents on the dollar raised was tied to development expenses. We are constantly weighing all of our expenditures for generating funds and have to look at the long-term perspective. For example, some of the current investment in our alumni will not pay off until 20 years from now.

Principle 12: Visibility is the key to success.

This visibility is important for students, faculty, and the administrative staff. We must participate in all of the community committees, the community activities that involve health care and that involve human services. Only when we are visible in the community will people want to invest in our academic programs.

Frequently asked questions and answers about fund-raising are as follows:

Q. What drives your fund-raising?

A. Strong academic programs, new programs and flexibility are important keys to our development success. In our strategic planning in the 5-year period prior to the campaign, a motto for our school—"a tradition of

innovation"—characterized our programs. It has served us well in launching new programs and in supporting all programs.

Q. What drives your collaborative relationships?

A. Strong academic programs, new programs, and flexibility in developing programs.

Q. What is the key to your development system?

A. Communication. We constantly communicate with everybody, whether they are previous donors from a foundation or a corporation, or whether they are current students who will be future alumni.

Q. What is the relationship between the School of Nursing's development effort and the university's development efforts?

A. Coordinated, requiring a great deal of communication. The coordination is necessary with the university because there are a number of professional schools interested in the same foundations and the same donors. Before we approach a donor, we must request clearance from the university's development office which acts as a clearinghouse. Two principles are used in making the decision for clearance: which is the largest gift and the closest relationship or the closest potential relationship.

Q. Do you employ your own staff?

A. Yes, we are a decentralized university so that each management center stands on its own. Therefore, we are totally responsible for

▲ ▲ ▲

It is a challenge to always

be there when the decision

is made. If you are not

there, if you don't have a

current relationship with

somebody you think has

the potential of supporting

your programs, then it is a

hard sell.

▲ ▲ ▲

generating our own funds for all of our programs. Whatever resources we generate, we can spend.

Q. How big is the development team in the School of Nursing?

A. We currently are finishing a campaign, so we are still staffed at our campaign level of four professional development staff and two support staff. In 1982, we had one half-time staff member assigned to development in the School of Nursing.

Q. Can you identify some potential audiences that could be targeted for a development campaign?

A. The immediate potential is for foundation support and individual support, knowing that the individual support takes longer to generate. There are a number of foundations—local, regional and national—committed to health care or new programs that address health care issues. There is much more potential for generating foundation support in health science schools. Piggyback on the successes of other institutions. Find out everything about what potential there is in the area. Find a good mentor. Relate to your local community. If the locals do not view

you as a star, then you will have a hard time getting national support.

Q. Of the monies that you talked about, what share was for endowment and what share was for operating revenue?

A. About a third of our campaign commitment was endowment support. We would have liked that to be 50%. Since 1982, our endowment has increased from $8 million to $27 million. Over the years we have purposely focused on generating endowment support because we believe that will put us in the best long-term position. Given a choice, we would always like to have endowment. It is often a struggle because you do have programs that you want to support, so it is a judgment call. Many foundations only give to operating and current program support. With the individual gift it is a hard judgment call, and I always lean on the side of endowment. If you have a situation where there is a current operating deficit, obviously it is important to get out of that deficit position before you can start building an endowment.

Q. What percent of your budget is from tuition?

A. Approximately 50%. In the last 12 years we have not varied much in our tuition as a percent of our overall revenues.

Q. In your relationship with the rest of the university with coordination, when you want to approach a major corporation, do you need to clear it within the university system so that everybody cannot approach at the same time?

A. Yes, and we have not always won, but we keep trying. In fact, it is a challenge to always be there when the decision is made. If you are not there, if you don't have a current relationship with somebody you, think has the potential of supporting your programs, then it is a hard sell. You have to build the potential relationship. I can give you a good example of that. We have a program that we have started in home care. I have to say that we invested in the program before it was clear that that was the direction in which the world was going.

I have summarized what I believe to be the common themes in all of the principles that I have noted which are these values: collaboration, communication and cooperation.

▲ ▲ ▲

Joyce J. Fitzpatrick, PhD, MBA, RN, FAAN, is Professor of Nursing and Dean of the Frances Payne Bolton School of Nursing at Case Western Reserve University, Cleveland, OH. Dr. Fitzpatrick is widely published in the nursing literature, having over 100 publications. She is coeditor of the Annual Review of Nursing Research *series and editor of* Applied Nursing Research.

▲

Appendix E

Fundraising Reports from the Council for Aid to Education

TOTAL PHILANTHROPY IN THE U.S.

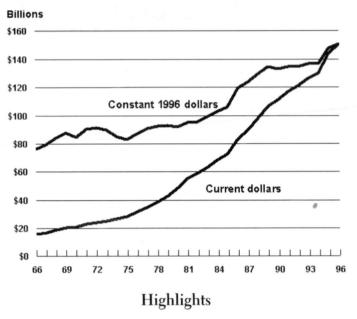

Highlights

- Total philanthropy, which includes charitable contributions from individuals (both living and through bequests) and from corporations and foundations, is estimated to have reached almost $151 billion in 1996, a 7.3% increase over the 1995 figure of $140 billion.
- In current dollars, there has been a ten-fold increase in total philanthropy over the past thirty years. In constant dollars, the picture is less dramatic, with total philanthropy doubling over the past thirty years, comparable to growth of Gross Domestic Product (GDP) during the same period.
- Contributions from living individuals (79.6%) and bequests (6.9%) together account for almost 87% of total philanthropy. Corporations (5.6%) and private foundations (7.8%) provide the remaining 13.4%. However, gifts to religion (almost all from individuals) account for 46 % of total philanthropy. Corporate and foundation giving accounts for 25% of total philanthropy when gifts to religion are excluded.

Notes

Constant dollars based on the Consumer Price Index (CPI).
Source: *Giving USA 1997*, AAFRC Trust for Philanthropy, 1997.
Copyright © 1997, Council for Aid to Education.

DISTRIBUTION OF TOTAL PHILANTHROPY BY CAUSE

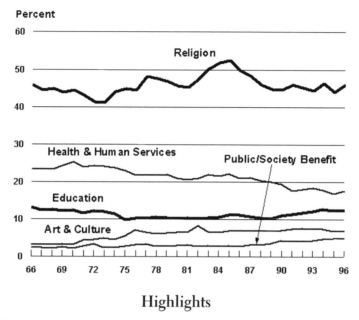

Highlights

- The relative standings of the different primary sectors have remained constant over the past 30 years. Religion receives the most—now at 46.1%, about its share 30 years ago. Some of the funds given to Religion ultimately find their way to causes reflected in the other categories.

- Health and Human Services is second—now at 17.3%. This category has experienced a gradual decline during much of the period charted.

- Education is third—now at 12.5%. Education's share has been rising since the late 1980s. Art and Culture is fourth—now at 7.2%. This represents a significant increase since the mid-1960s. Public/Society is fifth at 5% and has also been climbing slowly but steadily for the past decade.

- Other categories, not charted, account for the remainder. These include Environment/Wildlife, International Affairs, Gifts to Foundations, and Undesignated, which has fluctuated considerably over the years.

Notes

Source: *Giving USA 1997*, AAFRC Trust for Philanthropy, 1997.
Copyright © 1997 Council for Aid to Education.

TOTAL CONTRIBUTIONS TO HIGHER EDUCATION

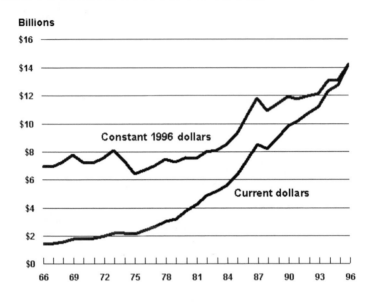

Highlights

- Total contributions to higher education from all sources reached an estimated $14.25 billion in the 1995–96 academic year. Included in this amount is giving from alumni, parents, other individuals, corporations, foundations, religious organizations, fundraising consortia, and other organizations (e.g., fraternal organizations and unions).
- There is the familiar growth curve—almost a ten-fold increase in current dollar support over the past 30 years.
- In constant dollars, support has more than doubled over the past 30 years.
- The major current dollar dip, in 1987-88, was due to a combination of the Tax Reform Act of 1986 and the stock market crash of 1987. But there was a return to the upward trend in 1988–89.
- Slow growth or declines during the 1969–71 and 1973–75 periods correspond to economic recessions.

Notes

Constant dollars based on the Consumer Price Index (CPI).
Source: *Voluntary Support of Education 1996,* Council for Aid to Education.

SOURCES OF SUPPORT OF HIGHER EDUCATION

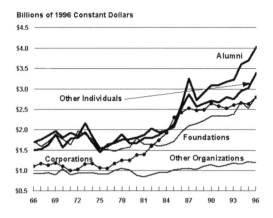

Billions of 1996 Constant Dollars

Highlights

- Note that Alumni and Other Individual giving bounced back in 1988–89 following the drop in 1987–88, a drop due to accelerated giving in advance of the 1986 Tax Reform Act and to the stock market crash of 1987.
- The corporate figures reported here tend to be larger than the corporate figures reported in earlier charts. The earlier charts reflect the outflow of contributions from corporations and their foundations, as reported by corporations, and are on a calendar year basis.
- Corporate giving figures reported on this and subsequent charts reflect the inflow of corporate dollars as reported by the educational institutions and are on an academic year basis. Educational institutions include (not necessarily inappropriately) in their corporate gift totals certain amounts that corporations account for outside of their contributions budgets; for example, human resources, research, public relations. There are also differences in the way corporations and educational institutions value gifts of product and property. Finally, educational institutions report corporate gifts received from corporations based outside the United States, while Council surveys of corporate contributions and estimates based on those surveys are limited to U.S.-based corporations.

Notes

Source: *Voluntary Support of Education 1996*, Council for Aid to Education. Copyright © 1997, Council for Aid to Education.

DISTRIBUTION OF CORPORATE CONTRIBUTIONS BY CAUSE

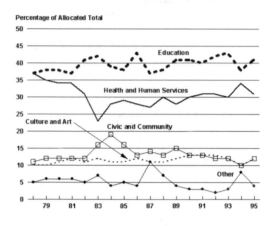

Highlights

- The percentage shares of allocated corporate contributions to beneficiary groups are based on responses to an annual survey of corporate contributions conducted by the Council for Aid to Education (conducted jointly with The Conference Board through 1994, with estimates for 1995 based on the average of the prior 5 years). The survey results should be taken only as generally indicative of the way all corporations in the aggregate probably distribute contributions to different causes.
- The choice of beneficiary group to which a gift is reported as going may be misleading. For instance, a contribution to a university medical center for medical research is properly reported as a gift to education since the check is made out to a university. But this is not support of education as commonly conceived. Nevertheless, basic corporate priorities are apparent and have maintained their relative standings over the period in question.
- The Council estimates that support of education, as a percentage of total consolidated corporate support by all corporations, currently stands at about 41%, a level to which it has risen from an estimated 36% in 1971. It is not expected to climb significantly beyond this level.

Notes

Source: Council for Aid to Education.
Copyright © 1997, Council for Aid to Education.

CORPORATE SUPPORT OF
EDUCATION — PERCENTAGES

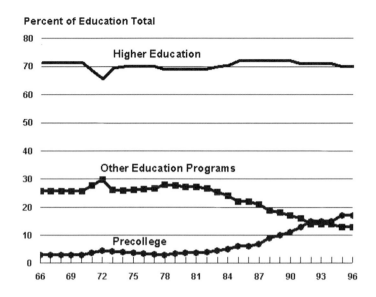

Percent of Education Total

Highlights

- Higher education is the major recipient of consolidated corporate support of education, and currently receives an estimated 70% of the education total. Perhaps 5% or more of the dollars going to higher education institutions have as their ultimate target elementary and secondary school support, improvement and reform.
- Other Education Programs (scholarships and fellowships, education-related organizations) now receive about 13% of the total. The Council estimates that about 80% of this 13% goes to higher education-related causes. The remaining 20% has a precollege focus.
- Precollege education is now estimated to receive about 17% of the total. Its share of the total began to grow in the late 1970s.

Notes

Source: Council for Aid to Education.
Copyright © 1997, Council for Aid to Education.

CORPORATE SUPPORT OF EDUCATION

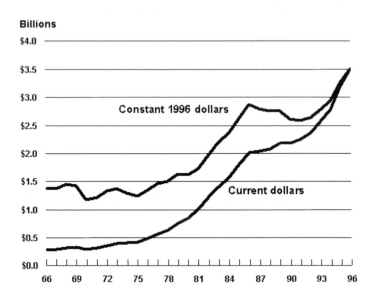

Highlights

- In current dollars, there has been more a twelve-fold increase in corporate support of education over the past 30 years.
- In constant dollars, contributions have grown over 2½ times over the past 30 years.

Notes

Constant dollars based on the Consumer Price Index (CPI).
Source: Council for Aid to Education.
Copyright © 1997, Council for Aid to Education.

ALUMNI SUPPORT OF STUDENTS

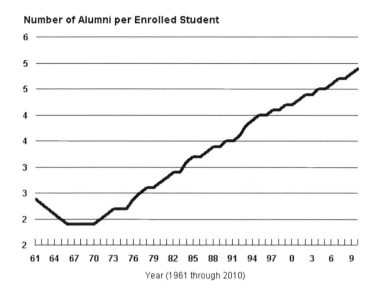

Number of Alumni per Enrolled Student

Year (1961 through 2010)

Highlights

- Enrollment (full- and part-time) grew 147% from 1961 to 1990. By the year 2010 it will only grow another 21% of the 1961 amount.
- Conversely, the alumni pool grew about 200% just between 1961 and 1984. By 2010 it will have grown 4.5 times the 1961 amount.
- Put another way, in 1961 there were 2.4 alumni for every enrolled student. A low was reached in the late 1960s of only 1.9 alumni per student. Since then the ratio has climbed to 3.5 and by 2010 the ratio will approach five alumni per student.

Notes

Source: Special study commissioned by the Council for Aid to Education ("Alumni Giving to the Year 2010," Prof. Ralph Bristol).
Copyright © 1996, Council for Aid to Education.

ALUMNI TOTAL, BASE, AND AVERAGE GIFT

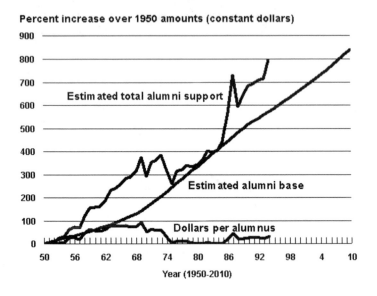

Percent increase over 1950 amounts (constant dollars)

Estimated total alumni support

Estimated alumni base

Dollars per alumnus

Year (1950-2010)

Highlights

- The significant growth in total alumni giving (constant dollars) over the past 40 years is largely a function of the expanding alumni base. The average gift per alumnus (in constant dollars) has changed little. But this is to be expected given the fairly constant age factor through the early 1980s and the poor performance of the stock market from the early 1970s to the early 1980s.
- As the alumni base continues to grow and mature, we should see robust increases in aggregate alumni support.

Notes

Constant dollars based on the Consumer Price Index (CPI).
Source: Special study commissioned by the Council for Aid to Education ("Alumni Giving to the Year 2010," Prof. Ralph Bristol).
Voluntary Support of Education 1995, Council for Aid to Education.
Copyright © 1996, Council for Aid to Education.

VOLUNTARY SUPPORT AS A PERCENTAGE
OF EXPENDITURES

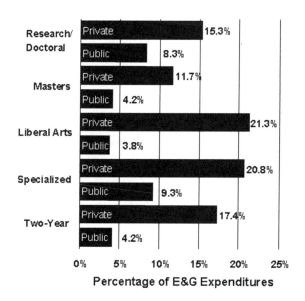

Percentage of E&G Expenditures

Highlights

- This figure shows, for the various types of higher education institutions, the relative significance of voluntary support as a percentage of Educational and General Expenditures.
- Within each Carnegie group, the private institutions are covering at least twice the percentage of expenditures as are the public institutions.

Notes

Source: *Voluntary Support of Education 1996,* Council for Aid to Education.

Copyright © 1997, Council for Aid to Education.

CORPORATE SUPPORT: PUBLIC AND PRIVATE INSTITUTIONS

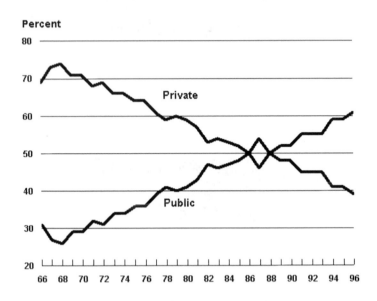

Highlights

- Culminating a long-term trend, total reported corporate support to private four-year institutions dropped below total reported corporate support to public 4-year institutions for the first time in 1988–89.
- These lines are based on survey results. We do not know whether corporate gifts to all public institutions together would exceed corporate gifts to all private institutions.
- Regardless, on a per-student basis the gap has not narrowed by nearly as much since public institutions have grown in number and size much more than private institutions over the past 20 years.

Notes

Source: *Voluntary Support of Education 1996*, Council for Aid to Education.

Copyright © 1997, Council for Aid to Education.

FOUNDATION SUPPORT PER STUDENT
BY TYPE OF INSTITUTION

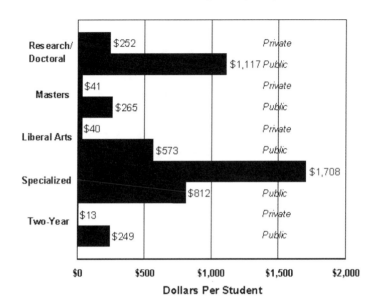

Highlights

- This chart shows the distribution of private foundation dollars by type of institution in the 1995–96 academic year.
- These figures are derived from survey results and are not estimates. Enrollment is measured by straight headcount, not full-time equivalent (FTE).
- If FTEs were used, the public average per student would increase, but not substantially.
- Note that there are very few students in the public specialized institutions (frequently medical schools and health science centers). So while the dollars per student are large, the total dollars to this type of institution are small.

Notes

Source: *Voluntary Support of Education 1996*, Council for Aid to Education.

Copyright © 1997, Council for Aid to Education.

DISTRIBUTION OF TOTAL GIFTS BY PURPOSE

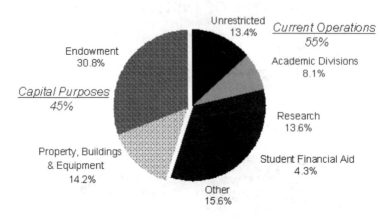

Highlights

- This chart shows the distribution of support from all sources by purpose for all higher education institutions participating in the 1995–96 Voluntary Support of Education survey.
- The Current Operations Other Restricted slice includes Faculty and Staff Compensation, Operation and Maintenance of Physical Plant, Public Service and Extension, Library, and Other Restricted Purposes.

Notes

Source: *Voluntary Support of Education 1996*, Council for Aid to Education.
Copyright © 1997, Council for Aid to Education.

DISTRIBUTION OF CORPORATE GIFTS BY PURPOSE

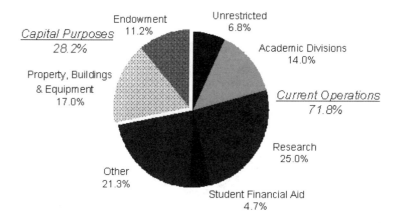

Highlights

- This chart shows the distribution of support from corporations by purpose for all higher education institutions participating in the 1995–96 Voluntary Support of Education survey.
- The Current Operations Other Restricted slice includes Faculty and Staff Compensation, Operation and Maintenance of Physical Plant, Public Service and Extension, Library, and Other Restricted Purposes. Much of the Property, Building & Equipment amount represents corporate gifts of product and property.

Notes

Source: *Voluntary Support of Education 1996,* Council for Aid to Education.

Copyright © 1997, Council for Aid to Education.

DISTRIBUTION OF FOUNDATION GIFTS BY PURPOSE

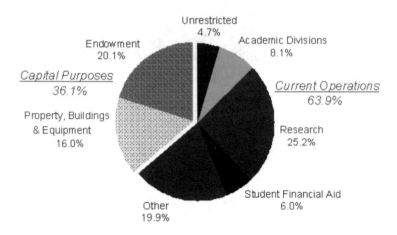

Highlights

- This chart shows the distribution of support from foundations by purpose for all higher education institutions participating in the 1995–96 Voluntary Support of Education survey.
- The Current Operations Other Restricted slice includes Faculty and Staff Compensation, Operation and Maintenance of Physical Plant, Public Service and Extension, Library, and Other Restricted Purposes.

Notes

Source: *Voluntary Support of Education 1996*, Council for Aid to Education.

Copyright © 1997, Council for Aid to Education.

SIGNIFICANCE OF LARGE GIFTS

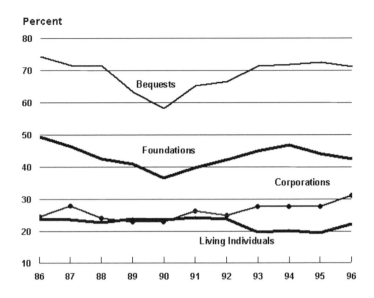

Highlights

- Institutions are asked to list their three largest gift totals from living individuals, from bequests, from foundations, and from corporations on the VSE Survey. These relatively few large gifts are of crucial importance.
- In 1996, the sum of the twelve large gifts to each of 1,078 institutions supplying complete information accounted for 35.2% (about the same as in recent years) of all the gift income reported by these institutions.
- The chart above shows the importance of large gifts for each of the four sources studied. As an example, the chart shows that in 1996 the sum of the 3 largest gifts from living individuals reported by each of the 1,078 reporting institutions equaled 22% of the total of all gifts from all living individuals reported by these institutions.

Notes

Source: *Voluntary Support of Education 1996*, Council for Aid to Education.

Copyright © 1997, Council for Aid to Education.

Index

Index

Accountability, 59, 65, 115
Acknowledgment letter, 93
Acknowledgments, donor recognition,
    114–116
"A Convergence of Interests," Case
    Western Reserve University
    activities, 105–106
    case statement, 104–105
    donors, pyramid of, 105
    leadership, 106
    motto, 105
    National Campaign, 106
    President's Weekend, 105–106
    public relations, 106–107
Advisory committee, 66–67, 97–98
Alumni Committee, 98
Alumni gift, case study, 119–120
American Association of Fund Raising
    Counsel (AAFRC), 8
American Council on Gift Annuities, 71
American Institute of Philanthropy, 141
Annual fund campaigns, 12, 24–26, 36
Annual Fund Committee, 98
Annual report, 116
Anonymous donors, 50, 65
Appointments, securing, 15–16
Appraiser, function of, 28
Art work, 29
Ask
    corporate development, 83–84
    minimum, 32–33
    size of, 18
Attorney, function of, 30, 86
Auctions, 36

Beliefs/values, perpetuation of, 41
Beneficiaries, 70
Bequests, 29–31, 37, 59, 69

Bill and Melinda Gates Foundation, 45
Board members, planned gifts from, 57,
    67
Briefing sessions, solicitation strategies, 19
Brochures, 60
Budget and Justification, 89–90
Building campaigns, donor recognition,
    40
Burnout, 100–101
Buy decision, 20

Calls for Proposals, 79, 87–88, 90
Campaign Committee, 99
Campaigns, case illustrations
    Case Western Reserve University,
        "A Convergence of Interests,"
        105–106
    School of Nursing Campaign,
        107–111
Capital gains, 70
Carnegie, Andrew, 7–8
Case statement, campaign, 104
Case studies
    alumni gift, 119–120
    gift of recognition, 121–123
    grateful patient, 120–121
Case Western University
    campaign case illustration, see "A
        Convergence of Interests," Case
        Western Reserve University Society
        of ENDOWMENTORS, 115
Cash gifts, 28
CEOs, planned gifts from, 67–68
Certificate of Deposit, 30
Challenge gifts, 26–27
Charitable intent, 67–68
Charitable lead trust, 73–74
Charitable remainder annuity trust, 72

Charitable remainder trusts, 70
Charitable remainder unitrust, 73
Chronicle of Philanthropy, The, 52, 79, 139–140
Closely held stock, 28
Collaborative fundraising, 2–5
Commitment
   to campaigns, 104
   planned giving programs, 59
   of volunteers, 96
   will, 30–31
Committees
   activities, 100
   advisory, 97–98
   alumni, 98
   annual fund, 98
   campaign, 99
   corporate, 99
   foundation, 99
   goals of, 99–100
   major gifts, 98
   purpose of, 97–98
Communication, importance of
   during campaigns, generally, 104
   during cultivation phase, 47–48
   in development process, 37
   donor recognition, 113–114
Community leaders
   cultivation of, 15–16
   planned gifts, solicitation of, 57
Concept Paper, 82, 87, 91
Confidentiality, 38
Connections, 141
Consultant(s)
   planned giving programs, 67–68
   role of, generally, 127
Contact, during cultivation phase, 48
Contact reports, 18
Contracts Weekly, 79
Corporate Committee, 99
Corporate development, see Grant-seeking
   decision makers, 86–87
   foundation distinguished from, 83
   gifts, 84
   information resources, 79–80
   leadership goals, 78–79
   partnerships, 81, 85

relationship building, 84–85
   targets, selection factors, 83, 85–86
Corporate Giving Watch, 79
Costs, for development, 126
Cost-to-benefit ratio, 36
Council for Advancement in Support of
      Education (CASE)
   contact information, 137
   as information resource, 142–144
Council for Aid to Education (CAE), 8, 38
Council on Foundations, 138
Counsel for Advancement and Support of
      Education (CASE), 116
CPA, function of, 66
Credibility, establishment of, 89
Cultivation phase
   grant-seeking and, 94
   overview, 15–16, 21, 35, 47–48

David and Lucile Packard Foundation, 45
Dean, perspectives of
   campaigns, 111–112
   cultivation, 17–18
   development office, staffing of, 131
   development officer, relationship with, 5–6
   gifting methods, 37
   individual gifts, 53
   reasons for giving, 43
   research, 13
   solicitation, 22
   stewardship, 118
   volunteers, 101
Debriefing, importance of, 35
Delegation, 5
Desire to belong, as motivation, 41–42
Development, basic principles of
   cultivation, 15–16
   dean's perspective, 13, 17–18, 22–23
   development officer's perspective, 12–13, 16–17, 22
   information resources, 13–14
   objections, answering, 21–22
   research, 11–12
   solicitation, 18–20

Development office
  consultant, role of, 127
  development officer's perspective, 130
  development professional, characteristics
    of, 127–129
  internal structures, 126–127
  staffing, 124–125
  success factors, 130
Development officer, perspectives of
  campaigns, 111
  cultivation, 16–17
  dean, relationship with, 5–6
  development office staffing, 130
  gifting methods, 36–37
  individual gifts, 49, 52–53
  on reasons for giving, 43
  research, 12–13
  solicitation, 22
  stewardship, 118
  volunteers, 100–101
Development professional, characteristics
    of, 127–129
Direct-mail campaigns
  effectiveness of, 34, 36
  Internet, 33
  length of appeal, 32
  minimum ask, 32–33
  packaging, 34
  personalized letters, 31–32
  special events and, 36
  text, 33
  time frame, 33
Discovery missions, 16
Donors, generally
  pyramid of, 105
  recognition of, see Donor recognition
Donor recognition
  methods/strategies, 113–115
  planned giving programs, 64–65
Dunlop, Dave, 57

Education, recent statistics, 8–9
Endowment funds, 42, 117
Endowment gifts, 20, 27, 30, 37
Estate planning, 21, 29–31, 69–71
Executive Summary, in proposal, 88, 90
Exit plan, 50

Face-to-face meetings, 48, 53, 61–62
Fair market value (FMV), 28, 58
Family foundations, 14
Family named gifts, 39–40
Feasibility studies, 67, 104
Feedback, importance of, 82, 101
501(c)(3) status, 90
Fixed income agreements
  charitable remainder annuity trust,
    72
  gift annuities, 71–72
Flexibility, importance of, 19, 78
Focus groups, as information resource,
    14
Follow-through, importance of, 129
Foundation, see Grant-seeking
  Application Guidelines, 87–90
  corporate development distinguished
    from, 83
  information resources, 79–80
  leadership goals, 78–79
  partnerships, 81
  Site Visit, 92–93
Foundation Center, The
  contact information, 138–139
  as information resource, 78–79,
    138–140
  publications, 139–140
Foundation Committee, 99
Foundation Directory, The, 80
Foundation Giving Watch, 79
Foundation Reporter, 80
Founder's Society, 25
Franklin, Benjamin, 7
Friend-raising, 46
Fundraising, generally
  basic principles of, 2
  experiences of, 2–5
  importance of, 1
  misperceptions of, 2

Gates, Bill, 8, 45, 49
Gates, William H., Jr., 45
Gift annuities, 70–72
Gift Club, 25
Gift of recognition, case study,
    121–123

Gifts, types of
  annual fund, 24–26
  bequests, 29–31
  challenge gifts, 26–27
  outright gifts, 28–29
  restricted gifts, 27–28
  unrestricted gifts, 27
Gift Table, sample, 135
Gift trees, 40
Giving, reasons for
  affinity to programs and goals of
    institution, 42
  commitment to give something back,
    40–41
  desire to belong, 41–42
  guilt, 42
  memorials, 39
  perpetuating one's beliefs, 41
  personal legacy, 39–40
  recognition, 40
GIVING USA, 44
Goals, identification of, 101
Government bonds, 28
Grant-seeking
  acknowledgment letter, 93
  applications, 87
  credibility, 89
  goals of, 78–79, 82, 94
  historical perspective, 76–77
  information resources, 79–80
  "lessons learned," 93
  meetings, preparation for, 82, 87
  participants in, 80–81
  partnerships, 81
  proposal, writing guidelines,
    see Proposals
  Site Visit, 92–93
Grateful patient, case study, 120–121
GuideStar, 140
Guilt, as gift motivation, 42

Health Care Grants, 79
High touch approach, 48, 62–63
Historical perspective, 7–8
Honor roll, 41–42
Humor, importance of, 129
Indebtedness, as reason for giving, 40–41

Individual gifts
  examples of, 45–46
  nurturing relationships, 51–52
  prospects, identification of, 46–47
  records, research and maintenance of, 51
  relationship-building, 47–50
Information resources
  CASE, 142–44
  grant-seeking, 79–80
  institutions and associations, 137–140
  Internet resources, 79–80, 87, 140–141
  on prospects, 13–14
  software resources, 141
  types of, 13–14
Institutions, gifts to, 31, 42
Internet
  direct-mail campaigns, 33
  as information resource, 79, 87
Irrevocable charitable trust, 58
Irrevocable gifts, 70
IRS Forms
  Form 990, 14
  Form 990-PF, 78

Legacy, personal, 39–40
Legal counsel, functions of, 27–29
Length of appeal, 32
"Lessons learned," 93
Letters, in direct-mail campaigns, 31–32
Letters of Support, 90
Life-income agreements, 70–71
Life insurance policies, 28, 74
Life insurance sales person, function of,
    66
Listening skills, importance of, 48, 128;
    see also Communication

Major campaigns, 125
Major donors, 47–48, 51
Major gifts, 48s, 59, 98
Major gifts committee, 98
Management skills, in development
    professional, 128
Marketing
  equation/exchange, 18
  planned giving programs, 57, 59, 62–64
Matching gifts, 26–27

McCarty, Oseola, 44–45, 49–50
Meetings
    planned gift programs, 61–62
    preparation for, 125
    with prospects, 48, 53
    securing appointments, 15–16
    site selection, significance of, 19
    with volunteers, 95–96, 100
Memorial gifts, 20, 39
Mini-campaigns, 103
Misperceptions, 2
Mission, 67–68
Mottos, 105
Moves Management approach, 57
Multiyear total giving, 115
Municipal bonds, 28
Mutual funds, 28

National Charities Information Bureau,
    140
National Committee on Planned Giving,
    68, 140
National Society of Fund Raising
    Executives (NSFRE), 68, 129,
    137
Networking, 77, 101
Newsletters
    foundation/corporate development,
        79
    planned giving programs, 63–64
Nightingala, 35, 109
Nonverbal communication, importance
    of, 19–20, 50
Nurturing relationships, 51–52

Objections, answering, 21–22
One-person office, 130
Open-ended questions, 21, 49
Operating plan, planned giving programs,
    65–66
Organization skills, importance of, 128
Outright gifts, 28–29, 37

Part-time fundraisers, 125
Payable on Death (POD), 30
Peer volunteers, 16
Personalized letters, 31–32

Personal visits, cultivation activity, 15–17,
    48
Philanthropic Advisory Service of the
    Better Business Bureau, 141
Philanthropic lifestyle, 61–62
Philanthropy
    education, recent statistics, 8–9
    historical perspective, 7–8
    schools of nursing, 9–10
Philanthropy, 139
Phone-a-thons, 34, 84
Planned giving, generally
    advanced issues in, 66–69
    bequests, 69
    fixed-income agreements, 71–72
    instruments/methods of, overview,
        69–75
    life-income agreements, 70–71
    life insurance, 74
    program development, see Planned
        giving programs
    real estate, 74–75
    significance of, 55–56
    success factors, 55–56, 58–59
    variable income agreements, 72–74
Planned giving officer, job description, 56
Planned giving programs
    advisory committee, 66–67
    consultants, working with, 67–68
    development of, 58–59
    donor recognition, 64–65
    establishment of, 60–61
    evaluation of, 66
    marketing, 57, 59, 62–64
    mission and charitable intent,
        68–69
    operating plan, drafting guidelines,
        65–66
    professional, generally, 58
    staffing, 61
    success factors, 58–59
Pooled income funds, 70, 72–73
President's Society, 25
Principal Investigator, 77, 90
Professorships, 117–118
Promotional materials, 60–61, 106–107
Property, transfer of, 29–30

Proposals
  acknowledgment letter, 93
  attachments, 89–90
  Budget and Justification, 89–90
  credibility, establishment of, 89
  Executive Summary, 88, 90
  internal review of, 91
  objectives, 89
  presentation of, 92
  submission of, 91
  writing guidelines, generally, 88–89
Prospect(s)
  base, 24
  giving potential, factors of, 12
  identification of, 46–47
  information resources, 13–14
  personal history of, 50
  research on, generally, 12, 15

Radio campaigns, 67
Real estate agent, function of, 66
Real estate gifts, 74–75
Receipts, 116
Recognition, as reason for gift, 40
Recognition plan, 42; see also Donor
  recognition
Record-keeping system
  establishment of, 126
  research and maintenance of, 51
Recruitment, of volunteers, 96
Relationship-building, 47–50
Rephrasing techniques, 22
Research, importance of, 11–12; see also
  Information resources
Residuary estate, 69
Restricted gifts, 27–28
Revenue enhancement, 117–118
Revocable gifts, 37
Rockefeller, John D., 7
Rockefeller, John D., Jr., 7
Role-play exercises, 19

Scholarship funds, 20, 27, 117
School of Nursing Campaign, campaign
  case illustration
  campaign activities, structure of, 108
  campaign budget, 109–110

Corporate Committee, 108
  informational pieces, 107–108
  Major Gifts Committee, 108
  Physician's Committee, 108
  Special Projects Committee, 109
  wrap-up and celebration, 110–111
Schools of nursing, historical perspective,
  9–10
Screening groups, as information
  resource, 14
Securities, 28
Seminars, 68
Shotgun approach, 77
Site Visit, 92–93
Solicitation
  Annual Fund campaigns, 25–26
  direct-mail campaigns, 33
  guidelines for, 18–20, 22
  of individual gifts, 49–50
Special events
  auctions, 36
  cost-to-benefit ratio, 36
  cultivation, 35
  effectiveness of, 34
  follow-up to, 35
  keepsakes/momentos, 35
  preparation for, 35
  stewardship, 117
Special societies, donor recognition,
  113–114
Sponsorships, 35–36
Staffing
  development office, 124–125
  planned gift programs, 61
Stalled solicitation, 5
Stewardship, see Donor recognition
  communications, 117
  effective, 50, 94, 113, 118
  personalized, 115
  special events and, 117
Stewardship letters, 117
Stock warrants, 28
Stocks, publicly traded, 28
Surveys, as information resource,
  14, 61
Taxation
  charitable remainder trusts, 70

family foundations, 14
receipts, 116
Telephone calls, *see* Phone-a-thons
    Annual Fund campaign, 26
    cultivation activity, 15, 17
Testamentary trust, 30
Thank-you notes, 114, 116
Third parties, individual gifts and, 49
Tickler reports, 117
Tokens, of donor recognition, 116
Top executives, cultivation of,
    15–16
Transfer on Death (TOD), 30
Trusts
    charitable lead, 73–74
    charitable remainder, generally,
        70
    charitable remainder annuity, 72
    charitable remainder unitrust, 73
    irrevocable charitable, 58
Turner, Ted, 8, 45

University Programs, 140
Unrestricted gifts, 27

Variable income agreements
    charitable lead trust, 73–74
    charitable remainder unitrust, 73
    pooled income funds, 72–73
Vision, importance of, 47
Volunteers, *see* Committees
    initial meeting with, 95–96
    number of, 67
    peer, 16
    planned giving advisory committee,
        66–67
    potential contributions of, 101–102
    roles of, 95–96
    selection factors, 96, 102
    treatment of, 97

Wills, *see* Bequests
Winthrop, John, 7